Thin Ever After:

The ten secrets to achieve your perfect weight… and happily keep it forever

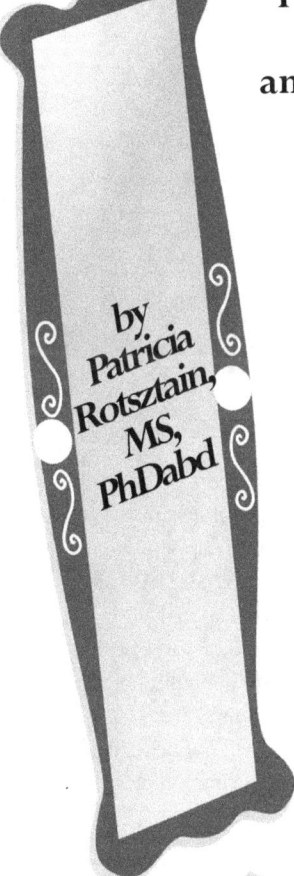

by
Patricia
Rotsztain,
MS,
PhDabd

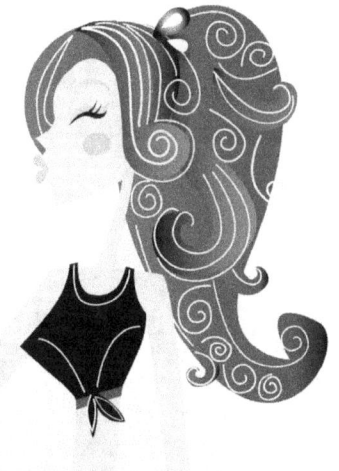

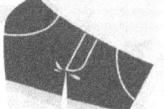

Preface

I am forty-six years old, about to be a grandmother, and still have the same weight I had when I was eighteen—124 pounds. I am not a Martian. I do not have iron will power. I've had break-ups and financial struggles, challenges and disappointments, and PMSing, just like you. I share 99.9 percent of my genetic makeup with the rest of human kind, including you. It's true, my metabolism is great, but *I* make it that way. And *you* can make it too, once you have the proper tools. That's what this book is about: the psychological and physiological tools you need to have the body you want and to feel good. This book will show you how to make peace with your hormones and enlist them as allies instead of sworn enemies, how to go from overeating to satisfaction, how to use your chemistry in your favor, and how to understand your emotions instead of numbing yourself with food. No more yo-yo diets, no more torture, no more fake promises that leave you disappointed and depleted. Instead, I propose you start truly inhabiting your body in joy by taking proper care of yourself with this simple system that lets you stop dieting and start making choices. Imagine yourself walking on the street, suddenly catching a glimpse of yourself in a store window, and feeling a warm sense of happiness as you smile at what you see… If you like the idea, go on reading and start melting excess fat, reshaping, detoxing, and feeling great… *Ever After.*

Acknowledgements

To my children, Luli and Tomas, who amaze me with their courage and
capacity to love, and who are wise beyond measure
and fill my life with joy and meaning.

To my mother, Perla, my cosmic companion who taught me to laugh,
even in the face of hardship.

To my unborn granddaughter, Anabella,
who makes my wrinkles worth it.

To my husband Joel, who respects my time and supports me
even when he doesn't fully agree.

To my brother, Danny, who looked at death in the eyes and made peace
with her; and who, by finishing his own book,
inspired me to do the same.

To my friend Adriana, who has relentlessly nagged me to write.

To G'd, who is a Genius!

To my angels, including Paulina

To Ella, who suggested the idea to go back to school
and follow my passion.

To my mentors, who have shown up in the form of books: Irvin Yalom,
Milton Erickson, Carl Jung, Clarissa Pincola Estez, Bruno Bettelheim,
Don Miguel Ruiz, and many others.

To my readers, who complete the circle I started.

Introduction

S andra was a princess born in Superland. Her parents were so excited about the birth of their firstborn and heir to the throne that months before her arrival they started planning the celebration party. And you can imagine what a celebration in Superland is like—land of the superbig, superfast, supersized. The queen hired Mr. Fancyshmancy, world famous designer to re-decorate the palace for the event and prepare the baby's chambers. Troops of chefs and their assistants, and their assistants' assistants moved in to start working on what would be the most exquisitely mouthwatering banquet in the history of Superland. Fairies and godmothers were diligently designing their gifts according to the traditions of the reign.

And the big day arrived...the cute round little baby came to the world. The celebration was nothing short of super. Thousands of guests paid tribute to little Sandra. Fifteen minutes before mid-night, the fairies and godmothers presented their gifts, as tradition dictated—a cell phone that would magically upgrade to the newest technology, so Sandra would always have the latest and never even have to ask for a new one; the "super outfitter," a computer program that would pick the perfect outfit for every occasion according to the latest trend, and materialize it; a carriage with sixteen white, winged horses that would take her anywhere and avoid traffic jams, equipped with video games and a large high definition screen; and so on and so on. The little princess received everything a girl could ever want...or did she not?

Well, it so happened that in a land of super-sizing, Sandra was not born with a genetic tendency to slimness. As the years passed, all those rich gourmet delights that were available at all times were piling up…around her thighs and belly. The aids and servants had been trained to anticipate to the princess wishes so she didn't have to move a finger to get what she wanted. As Princess Sandra grew up, all she wanted was to be thin. The queen and the king would desperately watch their daughter's despair as she became rounder and rounder. They took her shopping to distract her, but it only made things worse; nothing she liked would fit.

The princess would go on a strict diet, which she followed for a few days, until she would ravenously irrupt into the palace kitchen and devour every dessert and sweet in sight. So the king ordered the kingdom's wizard to create an artificial sweetener so that Sandra could lose weight without deprivation. It only made matters worse; it seemed that the pounds were glued to the princess forever. Then they ordered that any food prepared for the princess had to be absolutely fat free. Not only did the princess gain more weight, but now she was moody and depressed.

The years passed and Sandra was already in her late twenties. The time came when she was supposed to pick a spouse, but the princess would fiercely refuse to meet any of the suitors because she felt so miserable with her looks that she thought no one would possibly like her. The royal Wisdom Council was called for an emergency meeting. A solution had to be found so that the throne could be passed on according to the kingdom's traditions. The council's wise men were perplexed; they had never faced such a dilemma. Some anxiously played with their long white beards; others looked down in despair. A gloomy mood took over the large golden room. The silence was only interrupted by a nervous cough now and then. But suddenly, the doors opened, and all the eyes turned expectantly and shined with hope—the Green Fairy had arrived.

As she walked slowly and majestic in her green dress, sparks of stardust floating around her, the air filled with the fresh scent of mint and garden lilies. "There is one gift that the fairies did not give Princess Sandra at birth," she said. "In spite of my advice, the fairy's council voted against it because it was nothing spectacular. I have come today to correct the mistake and give her the missing gift, the antidote to excess, the solution to her problem. Without it, nothing can help her, not even the most illustrious expert. That gift, gentlemen of the Wisdom Council, is awareness, and it comes with a scale, a notebook, and a pen." A wave of "ohhhhhhhh" undulated around the table as the wise men moved their heads up and down. "In addition," the Green Fairy continued, "and in order to undo the damage caused, I am bringing this manuscript which, if followed, will make the magic work."

And this, my fellow seekers of the perfect weight, is the faithful transcription of the manuscript she carried in her hand— *Thin Ever After: The 10 Secrets to Achieve Perfect Weight, and Kept it Forever.*

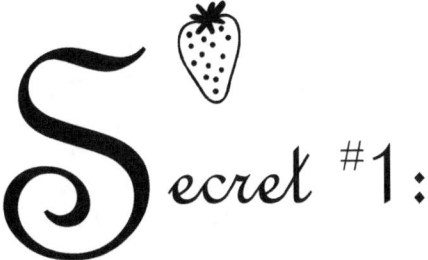

Secret #1:

The scale is not your enemy;
it's your copilot

Do you dread standing on the scale? Do you think that you don't need it because you can "tell by your clothes?" Well, my fellow seeker, you have to make peace with your scale. And if you don't have one, you need to get one now. The scale is your copilot, your companion in this journey. The scale doesn't lie to you. The scale gives you feedback on how you react to different foods or combinations and, like a good copilot, indicates which route goes to your destination.

You may be struggling right now to find excuses like "sometimes water retention may mask the real weight." That is precisely one of the feedback mechanisms that you need and that the scale provides. Water retention is a sign that something needs to be adjusted. It is not desirable, nor normal, to retain water within the tissues, to be bloated. Those are indications that your body disagrees with what you fed it. It may be that your protein intake is too low causing fluid to leak and get trapped in the spaces between the cells. It may be a sensitivity to a certain food that causes inflammation. Most people know when they are allergic to a food because they get an acute and immediate reaction they can connect to the food. If you are allergic to shellfish or peanuts, you will react right away. Food sensitivities, on the contrary, are not that cut and clear. Your body may take twelve to twenty-four hours to complain, and when it does, it won't be something spectacular, but instead a minor discomfort like, let's say, bloating or water retention. You probably consumed a lot of different things during all those hours, so how can you know which one produced the reaction? I'll explain that later when we talk about offenders and saboteurs in Secret 6. Right now, let's say that the scale can show you that there has been a saboteur. What good is a friend that lets you go out with a roller in your hair because she doesn't have what it takes to point it out? Why do you need a friend that lets you buy an outfit that doesn't fit because she doesn't want to hurt your feelings? The scale is your honest friend, the one that doesn't lie to you or act as a people pleaser, a friend that loves you so much that she will show you in numbers when you are on track and when you are not, the one that is not afraid to show you the truth. And, as Sigmund Freud once said, "The truth will set you free." He forgot to add that first it may piss you off.

Research shows that people that check their weight daily are much more successful at maintaining their weight loss. From the moment you start your weight loss plan, you are already in maintenance. You want to maintain every bit of success, don't you? I never understood those diets that have one, two, or three phases and *then* maintenance. Maintenance starts on day one. You want to maintain your new healthy changes and make them habits. You want to maintain any good result that you achieve. You want to maintain your motivation and determination for the rest of your life and from the first moment. So, if you have hidden your scale, go check your closets, basement, or attic and take it out. Hug it, make peace with it, and go put it back in your bathroom. Realize it is your friend and copilot and if it doesn't show you what you want to see, you need to change something, not hide it. Weigh yourself every morning when you wake up without clothes, and you will be part of that "much more successful" group that research shows. Neat, isn't it?

If you are thinking that you don't need the scale because you can tell by your clothes, keep in mind that, so far, your feedback mechanism hasn't worked that well. Unless you wear really tight clothes, which most people with excess weight don't do, by the time you notice it, you have gained quite a few pounds, usually more than five. If, on the contrary, you use the scale, and you notice you went up one or two pounds, it's easy to refocus and reverse the damage. If you were driving on a highway in the wrong direction, wouldn't you want to know as soon as possible so that you can turn around? Why would you want to wait until signs are written in a strange language?

You have probably tried many diets. You have probably regained the weight lost and even some more. Why not do things differently now? Remember, insanity is doing the same thing over and over and expecting a different result. Open your mind and give the scale a chance to help you. Besides, when you start practicing the *Ten Secrets*, the scale will give you good news. You will be thrilled to see the numbers go down. You will become aware of what makes them move faster or plateau.

You need to have the courage to accept where you are now. You cannot change what you don't know, what you ignore, or refuse to look at. As with any goal, you need to be realistic with both the starting point and the destination. You need feedback to adjust the plan. No journey is a straight line, so you will be permanently adjusting the steering wheel according to the turns and bumps in the road. This does not mean that the scale is the only feedback mechanism you have. The way you feel, your energy level, your mental clarity, the quality of your sleep, your resistance to disease, and your capacity to recover from it are all excellent indicators of your condition, of how well your food is nourishing and supporting your body. It is, however, not as clear or definite. Most of us have trouble giving those indicators a numeric value or noticing the subtle differences. We are not used or trained to ask ourselves how our mood has changed a few hours after a meal. Do we feel lethargic, foggy, edgy, irritable? If we do, how many times do we make the connection with the food that caused it? Each of these indicators is an important piece of information, and the fact that we add the scale does not invalidate or diminish the importance of the others. The more information we have, the easier it will be to make adjustments and keep on track. We need all of them. And how you can you make the best of them is to use them in synergy. Keep a journal of your daily weight, what and how much you ate, the circumstances when you ate, and make a note of your mood and energy level between meals. Here is an example of what it could look like for a typical female:

Tuesday.

Sleep: slept well, 7.5 hours
weight: 143 pounds

8 a.m.: 2 scrambled eggs with ½ cup of Fiber One, parsley and cilantro, 1 tbsp green powder drink in a glass of water; alone, at home

Between meal notes: high energy, focus, good mood

12 p.m.: salmon nicoise salad with olive oil and lemon, diet soda, coffee with cream, half apple pie portion; restaurant, with co-worker

Between meal notes: irritable, tired, moody, bloated

4 p.m.: ¼ cup of raw walnuts and one green apple; at desk, break.
Between meal notes: mood improved, more calm

6 p.m.: 1 chicken breast cooked in white wine and vegetable broth with onions and asparagus, ½ sweet potato, chamomile tea; home, with family.

    This kind of journaling can give you very valuable information. In this example, breakfast had a good combination of fat, protein, and carbohydrates. There were no caffeine or artificial stimulants. Instead, the natural energy of the green powder drink with spirulina and greens created a mood and energy level in the morning that was steady and good. In contrast, although lunch had a good main course, it also had a lot of caffeine, artificial sweeteners, and sugar. A few hours later the mood was irritable and the energy level low. The sugars and caffeine not only affected mood, but also interfered with digestion, causing a heavy and bloated feeling. The afternoon snack contained a good energy pick me up from the apple, plus the omega-3 good fats of raw walnuts, which worked together to help correct the previous imbalance and improve mood, leading to a good dinner choice. Had she instead had a candy bar or pretzels with more coffee, the negative cycle would have continued with more irritability, followed by a crash in energy, and more cravings.

By analyzing the food journal, we can clearly see which foods had a negative effect on this woman and which helped her feel good. The same will be true for our own journals. Over time, we will start to see patterns and detect the foods that cause sensitivity, impair digestion, and cause bloating. You may find out that you do perfectly well with fruits in the morning or between meals, but you get bloated if you eat them after meals. Or you may find you feel better if you eat one fruit at a time instead of mixing many. You may realize you do well with almonds butter but not with peanut butter. You'll find out differences in your sleep that will teach you what dinner choices help you sleep through the night and which cause you to wake up or toss and turn for hours. Maybe you do well with meat at lunch and not at night, or vice-versa. We are all different and there is not a one-size-fits-all diet. There are guidelines and information that will help you build the basics, but you will need to adjust and make changes that best suit your individual preferences and physiology. The scale will tell you each morning another side of the story. If you made good choices the previous day, your mood and energy level was balanced, and you slept well, but the number in the scale went up, maybe you need to adjust the quantity you eat. Maybe you do well with a few almonds, but not with a full cup. Maybe too much brown rice, although much better than white bread, still causes your blood sugar to spike. Maybe you didn't eat enough protein. What would happen if on the next day you have the same foods but increase protein?

Your mood and energy tell you if the choices you made were good for you, if the combinations work. The number on the scale tells you if it supports your weight loss plan. Both are important; you want to be thin *and* feel good. This is not about just shedding pounds. It is about doing it in a way that improves the quality of your life, your health, the way you feel. You can lose weight by drinking coffee and eating microwave packaged foods. But how will you feel? If a diet makes you physically weak and emotionally miserable, it will never work as a long time strategy. Your body, and rightly so, will react and rebel. But when instead, you find your match, that way of eating that fits you like a glove and helps you feel your best and improves your life, that is something you can willingly sustain for life. A scale, a notebook, and a pen—that is all the technology you need to be happily Thin Ever After!

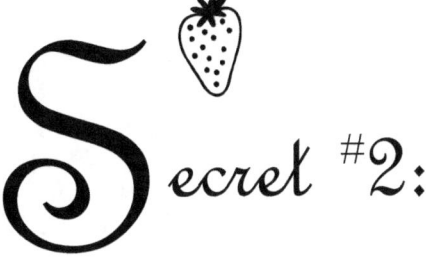

Secret #2:

Exercise. . .your right to be fit

The only predictor of good aging is the absence of a sedentary lifestyle. According to John Medina, author of "Brain Rules," exercise improves fluid intelligence and memory, cuts your chances of having Alzheimer's by 60 percent and stroke by 57 percent. It further reduces the risk of over a dozen cancers and diabetes, improves the immune system, regulates appetite, improves blood lipids, and makes your bones stronger, helping you prevent osteoporosis.

What good is having something that you cannot reach or use? By improving your supply of oxygen and quality of blood vessels, exercise allows your body better access to nutrients and better ways to dispose of waste.

As humans, we developed in movement. Our primitive ancestors walked about twelve miles per day. The calories spent in order to obtain food were in balance with the calories consumed with that food. We are designed to move. When we stop exercising and adopt a sedentary lifestyle, we are telling our brain that we are old, and that's what we get—we start getting old. And with old age, our metabolism slows down.

We've all heard it: "Exercise helps you lose weight and stay fit." Tons of research show very clearly that exercise has innumerable health benefits. Now how exactly does exercise help in your perfect weight dream? Is it because of the calories you burn? You will be surprised to know that the answer is maybe yes, and maybe no.

I work with many women that spend an hour a day running or take spin classes. They probably burn between 500 to 700 calories in that hour. Nice, isn't it? And it would be so if it weren't for the fact that they often believe that since they have exercised so diligently, they now "deserve" a reward. "I was such a good girl," they tell themselves, "I now deserve an ice cream, or a dinner at that Italian restaurant with the garlic rolls and the Alfredo pasta." At the end of the day, they burned 500 calories, consumed 500 in the ice cream or 1500 in the Italian restaurant dinner, and the next day weighed more than before; they are plus bloated and filled with toxins. Then they mourn and complain about how they "kill themselves" at the gym and still can't shed a pound.

Exercise works by increasing your metabolism, the rate at which you burn calories for energy. It also helps you flush cortisol, the stress hormone, out of your body. It helps manage stress (when you exercise you seldom think about stressful things). Sweating activates the largest detox organ in your body—your skin—so that you get rid of some of the toxins. Aerobic exercise strengthens your heart and lung capacity. Strength training or working your muscles using weights, machines, or just your own body (like in Pilates) builds muscle. Muscle, in turn, burns more calories than fat, so you not only look better (a toned firm butt rather than flan), but also boost your metabolism. Your bones benefit big time as well. Studies show that exercise is one of the best ways to prevent osteoporosis.

All these benefits are certainly desirable, but never an excuse to eat junk. What's the purpose of engaging in something with so many benefits just to ruin it at the end?

Many women ask me "What is the best form of exercise?" I respond: "The one that you actually DO." I don't care what you chose; it has to be something you enjoy, or you won't sustain it over time. It is better to go for a nice walk with your dog every day, month after month, than to join an expensive gym, take three spinning classes, and never set a foot there again. Exercise is any form of movement; it doesn't even have to be "formal." Playing ball with your kids, dancing, swimming, walking, taking the stairs instead of the elevator...it all counts.

If you find that strenuous aerobic exercise makes you ravenously hungry, try yoga. Yoga builds strength, improves balance, and even more important, builds your awareness of muscle. By requiring that you breathe deeply and diaphragmatically, it builds a memory of relaxation and improves focus. It also requires that you pay attention to your posture, adjust it, coordinate your breath, and keep your balance. Who can think of your credit card debt or your meeting in the afternoon when your mind is so busy doing all this to hold your posture? Yoga develops an awareness of your body sensations, which transcends the class. When you learn to pay attention to your body, you can become aware of being full more easily, or of how real hunger feels as opposed to anxiety. Although aerobic classes may burn more calories, have you ever noticed that people who practice yoga tend to be slimmer? You will seldom find an overweight yoga person.

Maybe you are now telling yourself that it is not for you; you are more of an active kind of gal. You like the speed, the rush; slow is not your thing. If you are thinking this, think again. How has all the running and never stopping to reflect served you so far? How come you can't stay quiet and make contact with what is really going on inside? Why do you constantly seek noise and distraction? What are you scared of? Whatever you are scared of, that is precisely what you need to face, contact, process, and let go...before you can let go of the pounds.

Nobody improves or moves forward from their comfort zone. You need the discomfort to push you. That which causes discomfort will soon be mastered and become comfortable, and that's when you again face the choice of staying there or taking the next uncomfortable challenge and grow.

When I talked about choosing something that you like so you can sustain it over time, it doesn't mean that it will feel comfortable from the beginning. Learning to dance salsa or tango can be frustrating at first, but you still know deep inside if dancing is something that eventually will give you pleasure.

What are some of your excuses for not exercising? Let's look at the most common ones.

- **I don't have time.**

You *think* you don't have time to exercise. How are you going to make time for all those doctor's appointments when your body and mind start failing due to your sedentary lifestyle? Time is eternal. You have all the time in the world. It's just a matter of priorities— it's not just about fitting in your jeans without holding your breath; it's about how you want to spend the rest of your life. You have time to go to the dry cleaner, but you don't have time to exercise? You spend thirty minutes doing your hair, but you can't go for a walk? You watch TV or talk on the phone or have a few irrelevant meetings instead of moving your butt? Why is it that everything and everybody comes first on your list rather than you? If your best friend asked you for a favor that required thirty minutes, you would probably say yes and you don't hesitate in running like crazy to take your kids to soccer practice. Let me tell you this: You are more important than your best friend, and the best example you can set for your child is honoring your needs. I don't care how many guilt trips you have bought over time. Please read this carefully: You have the right to take care of yourself. You are important. You must come first on your list.

By taking the time to exercise or do something for yourself, you are giving those around you permission to love and care for themselves. A happy and healthy mom is the best gift you can offer your kids. On every plane, they tell you that if there is a problem with the oxygen, you must put your mask first and then help your kids. Why? Because if you pass out, you won't be too much help. And the same happens with the rest of your life. Unless you take care of yourself, you will not be present for your kids.

"Love your neighbor as yourself," says the Bible. It doesn't say to love your neighbor *more* than yourself. If you can do so many things for your boss, your kids, your spouse, your friends, and your mother, why not do at least the *same* for yourself? Do yourself a favor, and quit that job as hostess of Guilt Trip airlines!

- **It's boring.**

Do you remember playing as a little kid? All that running and jumping and stretching and rolling was so much fun at that time.

What has changed since then? Why is it boring all of a sudden? Is it possible that it may not be boring, and that you just became self-conscious and embarrassed of how you look when you are moving? Are you comparing yourself to others, and self-criticizing? When you were a kid, you didn't bother worrying if your cellulite would show when you jump. When you were a kid, you did not look at your watch to decide when you had enough. You were just freely having fun. It's time to go back to that approach and search for activities that reconnect you with joy. Find a friend to exercise with you. Take your other half for a walk after dinner instead of growing roots from your tush in front of the TV. Play and laugh; stop thinking about exercise as another chore. It was natural and fun when you were a child and it can still be so. Download audio books into your iPod or MP3 player and listen to them while you exercise. Audible. com is a great site where you pay a subscription and download an immense variety of books in audio. That way, as you exercise, you can catch up on all those books you want to read, but can't find the time to do so. Everybody likes to be told a good story!

- **I have some physical problem.**

There is always something that you can do. Swimming or water aerobics take the pressure of your body weight off, and are great even for back problems. Besides, I have not yet found a physical problem that doesn't get better with exercise. The elliptical machine works well for those with knee problems that cannot run. You can exercise sitting, standing, or even lying down. Talk to your doctor and ask for a list of exercises that are suitable for your condition. Like Nike puts it: "Just do it!"

Make a goal to exercise ten minutes every day. When you say you will exercise for forty-five minutes it is easier to come up with excuses—you are tired, you have so much to do, and so on. Now if instead you decide to exercise for just ten minutes no excuse is valid. Who doesn't have ten minutes? Who can't put up with just ten minutes? You will probably find more often than not that after the ten minutes have passed, you decide to go for a little more. After all, you are dressed and already there, and it was not that bad, why not a little more? Setting ten minutes takes the pressure and the obligation off. It is totally doable and in my experience, most people expand those ten minutes to two or three times as much, and actually enjoy it. And if you only do those ten minutes, you have accomplished your goal, you succeeded, you are not a failure, and there is no guilt. Success brings more success by building confidence. You are also getting into the habit of exercising, which is important in itself, regardless of the length of time. It takes three weeks to incorporate something as a habit. Give yourself three weeks, and once you have the habit, your unconscious mind will help you maintain it; it will almost be like in automatic drive.

Scheduling your exercise is very important. It makes it real. One thing is saying, "I am going to exercise...sometime." It's another to say, "I am going to exercise from 7:00 to 7:30 p.m. tomorrow." Now it is a measurable and realistic goal. Write it in your calendar and treat it with the respect you treat any other appointment with someone else. Remember, you are at least as important as someone else is.

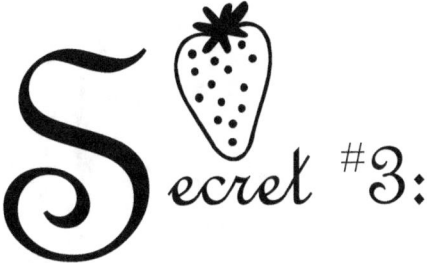

Secret #3:

Keep your cortisol in check.
Manage stress and sleep well

Stress

Being alive entails some degree of tension. Without it, you wouldn't be able to function. Stress is a necessary and normal part of life.

However, it is important to make a distinction between good stress and bad stress. Good stress is a low degree of tension that causes you to perform appropriately, and is motivating. Research shows that up to a certain point, stress enhances performance. When the level of stress passes a certain point, performance decreases accordingly, so the higher the stress goes up, the poorer performance becomes. A moderate amount of stress makes you feel awake, alive, engaged. Life situations that are considered "desirable" or "happy" can also be stressful—the birth of a child, moving, graduating, job promotions, or getting married.

The problem is that although we look very evolved and so-phisticated, and have machines, technology, cell phones, and other techno-chachkas, our brains are still wired in the same manner as the caveman's. Yep, it hasn't changed a bit. So, having that in mind, imagine that you are a caveman, thousands of years ago, and you venture outside to look for food, with your hide dress and your stick. You start walking, and a few minutes later…you find a lion in front of you—fierce, hungry, ready to attack. You know the only two options are to fight or run away. So your brain enters the "fight or flight response" and shuts down every system in your body that might take precious energy. You need all of it for this emergency; it's a life or death situation. Your immune system shuts down, your digestive system shuts down, (that's the dry mouth of fear), you start pumping cortisol and adrenaline, your heart starts beating fast, and your blood vessels constrict causing a rise in arterial pres-sure. Breathing becomes short and fast to provide extra oxygen to the rapidly circulating blood, and to give you an extreme state of alertness. An increased amount of glucose, or sugar, goes into the bloodstream to energize crucial muscles and organs. Your pupils di-late, to allow a better view. Voiding the body of digestive processes and waste material further prepares the organism for concentrated action, so there's a need to urinate or defecate, even vomit.

These unpleasant reactions were necessary to survive. Those humans that were able to produce this reaction were the ones that had better chances of surviving dangerous situations, and they passed their genes to us. That's what allows us today to lift a car in order to save a child, or exercise unusual and extreme strength in an emergency.

Let's go back to our caveman scenario and imagine you were lucky enough to survive. You probably burned up to a thousand calories in the event, either running away or fighting for your life. Food is difficult to find in these primitive times and although it's not easy to recover those lost calories, there is danger to your survival unless you can do that. So cortisol signals your body to make you ravenously hungry and hold on to every morsel of food, storing as much energy (calories) as possible.

Now, we live in funny times, where it is most improbable that we will confront a wild beast. However, we often have to confront a "wild boss" or client, or situations in which we perceive danger from a different source—danger to our job stability, our marriage, of not closing a transaction, of getting to the airport late and missing the plane, and so on. For our brain, it doesn't matter if it's a lion or an angry client, or the IRS—danger is danger, period. The physiological reaction is still the same…with one added peril. The caveman who fought or ran away consumed the adrenaline and glucose in his bloodstream. Nowadays, we no longer get into a physical fight (at least I hope you don't), nor do we run. But the mechanism works and cortisol still flushes our system. We stay still, so the chemical and physiological changes take much more time to normalize, with a very high cost to our health. We no longer expend the thousand calories, but we still crave the comfort foods and get this driving push to eat after a stressful episode. Have you ever craved an apple after being stressed? Most probably, you think of cookies, ice cream, or comfort foods…not fruit.

If your options were a coronary problem, stomach ulcer, extra pounds, or being devoured by a lion, you'd take anything but the last one. But is it worth having a stroke or becoming overweight for work related stress, traffic jams, or a nagging spouse? I don't think so.

Now that I have really started to depress you…I have good news: You can take action to change this. It is not possible for most of us to avoid stressful situations—at least I am not considering a Tibetan retreat life. Still, it is possible to counteract the effects of stress. To bring our bodies back to normal immediately in order not to build up. And that is what I propose to you today. Don't try to avoid stress (I am a hypnotherapist, not a magician), rather try to manage it, to control the effect.

The first step to managing stress is to recognize it. How many times do we not realize we are carrying tension in our neck and shoulders until we feel pain? How many times do we hold our jaws pressed without noticing until we have a headache? In order to recognize stress, we need a point of comparison with a non-stress state, that is, relaxation. We need to become familiar with being relaxed so we can recognize the difference between the two states. Now, an added bonus...learning to relax serves a dual purpose. It allows you to recognize bad stress, and it cure it—beautiful!

I want to remind you of a simple, fast, available resource that really, really works the minute you start using it. What I am going to give you is something you've always had—your breath. Your breath is a powerful link between your body and your mind. When you are stressed, or anxious, or have fear, your breath is short, fast, and shallow. When you are relaxed, your breath becomes slow and deep. You cannot be anxious, afraid, or stressed and relaxed at the same time. It is physically impossible. You cannot be stressed and breath slowly and deeply. It just can't happen. Why? Because there is a connection between your breath and your brain; that's the way it's wired. Think about it, you are on vacation sitting in a comfortable chair at the beach—it's the right temperature, you can smell the Hawaiian Tropic on your skin, there's a nice breeze, you hear the sound of waves, you're almost about to fall asleep into a delightful nap. How's your breath? Slow and deep. It goes along with that mindset.

The beauty of this is that if you are stressed there are two things you can do to get you closer to a state of relaxing on the beach. You can either think pleasant relaxing thoughts and slow your breath, or you can change your breathing and, thus, change your mental state.

To regulate your breathing, you can be standing or sitting, even walking, with your eyes open or closed, although we will start with eyes closed first. The whole purpose of *slow diaphragmatic breathing* is to have the exhalation longer than the inhalation. The inhalation part of the breathing cycle is the energizing part; it activates the sympathetic system, the arousal system, while the exhalation is the relaxing part, acting on the parasympathetic system, the part of the brain in charge of calming and curing the effects of stress. So, by extending the exhalation phase, you are relaxing your body and calming your mind.

We normally take twelve to thirteen breaths per minute. That's approximately one every five seconds. When you inhale, your heart rate actually increases a few beats per minute and your blood pressure goes up slightly. When you exhale, your heartbeat slows down and your blood pressure actually drops a few millimeters. By prolonging your exhalation, besides breathing more slowly, you are slowing down your heart rate and reducing your blood pressure. So by practicing slow deep breathing on a regular basis, you are calming down your heart and your autonomic nervous system as well.

Before you start this activity, you need to be able to recognize deep breathing. Most people, when asked to breath deep expand their upper chest, which feels most uncomfortable. So, put your left hand on your chest and your right on your abdomen. When you inhale, your abdomen goes out, pushing your right hand. When you exhale, your abdomen goes in, and so does your right hand. Your left hand doesn't move. You want to aim for a four-second to eight-second count. That means you will count to four when inhaling, and count to eight when exhaling. If that doesn't feel comfortable, adjust it to your own need (e.g., try three to six until you are familiar and then four to eight). Remember, this is not a competition or marathon; it's relaxation.

You want to do three to five rounds, or cycles, ten times a day and one five-minute session at night before going to sleep. The reason is that you want to build a memory of relaxation. The more you practice it, the more it works when you need it. It takes about three months to learn a new behavior pattern. Since you may have been breathing in a non-relaxing pattern for years you can't change it overnight, nor by doing it once in a while. Trust me; this is cheaper than Paxil—no prescription needed, always available, and no harm to your sex life!

Sleep

Now, let's take a look at how sleep affects our weight. Being fit is all about balance. That's why movement, action, and exercise need to be balanced with rest, and not just any kind of rest, but a good night's sleep.

you don't sleep the amount of hours you need (seven to eight hours, depending on age), your body's temperature the next day is lower. In an attempt to bring your temperature back to normal range, your brain pushes you to eat more, and usually craves foods that are higher in fats and carbohydrates. Every time you deprive yourself of sleep, you eat more and gain weight the next day. Studies show that people who sleep less than they need consume 15 percent more calories the next day.

We have a biological clock by which our metabolism and hormones run. Your immune system, sodium and potassium balance, blood sugar, body temperature, and repair mechanisms all are closely related to that biological clock. When your lifestyle doesn't synch with your biological clock, your health is negatively affected and so is your weight.

Sleep is closely related to cortisol levels in your body. Insufficient sleep forces your cortisol levels to rise. Please keep in mind the reason why cortisol was created. Cortisol, or "the stress hormone" was put into our system as a survival mechanism at the beginning of humankind. You may want to go back to the previous section on *Stress* if necessary. During the day, your cortisol levels are higher because you are faced with a variety of stressful instances, even if it is a traffic jam. When you sleep, your cortisol level is reset and goes down again. But when you don't sleep enough, your cortisol levels never go down and rise even further, making you hungry and quickening fat storage the next day, especially around your waistline. The average woman between thirty to sixty years old sleeps less than seven hours during the week. We need at least eight hours. So is there any wonder why we have trouble with weight?

Lack of sleep also affects other hormones, including growth hormone, which is needed to build lean muscle and reduce fat, so insufficient sleep not only makes you gain weight, but it is also responsible for the flabbiness.

In order to improve your sleep, start unwinding in the evening. Avoid difficult conversations at night, or watching the news. Don't exercise strenuously before going to bed, since it will wire you up. Instead, do things that are relaxing, like listening to soothing music, or taking a hot bath. Eat dinner at least two hours before going to bed. Make sure you have a good mattress and that your bedroom gives you cues for relaxing. A computer in your bedroom makes it hard to forget about work problems and tempts you to turn it on if you wake up during the night, something that will keep you up for hours. Once in bed, make a list of all the things you are thankful for. Even the worst days have something for which you can be thankful. Focusing on that will set the mood for peaceful sleeping. If your head keeps shooting thoughts and worries, visualize yourself gathering all those worries, or writing them down in a piece of paper. Then see yourself putting the worries or the paper with the list in a bubble and ask the universe to take care of them and watch them while you sleep. Take a few deep diaphragmatic breaths, and slide into a pleasant sleep.

If you wake up at night repeatedly, pay attention to the time. Chinese medicine states that the time you wake up has to do with certain systems in your body. When you consistently wake up between 11:00 p.m. and 1:00 a.m., your gallbladder may be involved. The gallbladder is in charge of carrying toxic waste in bile so it can be disposed of. If the bile is thickened by too many toxins, the gallbladder may get clogged and be unable to perform its job. It is necessary to keep the bile fluid and running. According to Chinese medicine, the gallbladder is related to the emotion of resentment. What are you resenting? Is there anything in your life you resent but are unwilling to admit? Are you constantly doing things for others but secretly feel used or abused? Do you resent the fact that others don't pay you back for all you do for them? Reflecting on this may bring this hidden feeling to the surface so you can accept it and process it, making the waking up unnecessary.

If you tend to wake up between 1:00 and 3:00 a.m., your liver may be complaining of too many toxins to filter. A cup of hot water with the juice of a fresh lemon first thing in the morning helps detox your liver. Also, certain herbs like milk thistle and supplements like alpha lipoic acid support the liver. Review your diet and get rid of chemicals and toxins as much as you can. A liver detox maybe a helpful step. Interestingly, Chinese medicine also says the liver is related to the emotion of anger. Are you repressing any anger that needs to come out and wakes you up at that hour? What are you angry about? What are you not contemplating or denying that produces anger? You may be surprised to find out that once you ask yourself these questions and take a look at your repressed anger, you won't wake up at night any more. Just becoming aware of it does the trick.

The hours of 3:00 to 5:00 a.m. are connected to the lungs. If you wake up at that time, you may want to check if there is any congestion present or respiratory difficulty. The lungs in turn are related to the emotion of sadness. Is there anything that makes you sad and you refuse to look at? Are you hiding your sadness or refusing to accept it? Are you repressing rather than working through your sadness? Again, just asking yourself these questions and becoming aware of your sadness and accepting it is enough to stop waking up.

Your waking up may be the way your body, or your subconscious, is trying to tell you something. Listen to them lovingly.

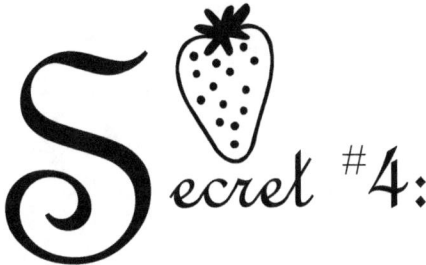

Secret #4:

Hormones rule

When Princess Sandra got her first period at thirteen, her world changed. Up to that moment, the king ruled over the kingdom, the moon ruled over tides, seasons ruled over crops. Once Sandra reached puberty...hormones ruled over EVERYTHING. The estrogen-progesterone balance is responsible for mood changes, water retention, fat accumulation, and pretty much all in a woman's world. When Sandra, and each of us, ovulates, we are getting ready for a potential pregnancy. Nature's pull is toward the survival of the species, rather than the fitting of the jeans. In an effort to ensure—should we get pregnant—that we have enough reserves stored to make that baby grow even in a famine, estrogen secretion increases and inhibits thermogenesis. Thermogenesis is the process of converting calories to energy or heat—in plain terms, fat burning. We gain fat, and that same fat produces more estrogen, which, in turn, produces more fat. Progesterone levels go down, increasing water retention. This "gift of nature" is supposed to go away once it is evident that we are not pregnant, and it becomes unnecessary. In some women, it lasts a few days and just means a couple of pounds fluctuation and a few days when clothes feel tight; then it goes away. But in others, like Princess Sandra, this cycle becomes permanent, and the weight gain from fat and water retention becomes permanent, adding up month after month. Also, estrogen levels remain high. This is called "estrogen dominance." Estrogen dominance causes fat to be stored in the waistline, thighs, and butt; water retention; and bloating. It also affects your body's production of serotonin by disrupting metabolization of an amino acid called tryptophan. As you probably know, serotonin is one of the "feel good neuro-juices" and its deficiency produces that blues feeling, cravings for carbohydrates and sugar, and an irresistible desire to jump at our mate's jugular like a crazy pit bull or snap at our best friend. If estrogen becomes much higher than progesterone, it can also affect the thyroid gland. This gland is responsible for telling the pancreas to produce insulin. When there is too much insulin in the bloodstream, you may get hypoglycemia, or low blood sugar, and then get intense irresistible cravings for carbohydrates and sugar.

When progesterone is too low, it doesn't have the strength to signal the hypothalamus to increase body temperature, so your metabolism becomes slow, like a furnace that has a tiny little flame, and cannot burn a lot of calories. If progesterone is too high, it increases appetite, food absorption, insulin, and the extra blood glucose becomes pounds of stored fat.

As you can see, this is a delicate balance, an orchestra where every hormone is an instrument that has to play in perfect synch for the music to be pleasant…and the jeans to fit.

Unfortunately, there are other added causes of hormone imbalance. Many medications we take, from birth control pills to some common cold medicines disrupt this balance. Non-steroid anti-inflammatory drugs, corticosteroids, blood pressure and diabetes medication, tranquilizers, and sleeping pills all affect hormonal balance. Please, under no circumstance, stop taking any of these medications on your own because what you just read freaked you out. This is just meant for you to be aware and explore, with your doctor, other more natural options and alternatives. Look for a doctor that is trained in both sides of medicine, mainstream and holistic. There are many natural herbs and therapies that may make it possible to reduce or eliminate the use of drugs. Ultimately, it is up to you to evaluate the cost and medical benefit. Now that you know how this works, you may decide that it is worth reducing salt and beginning exercise rather than taking a high dosage of a drug. Or, you may have an epiphany and realize that it may make sense to go to therapy and work through your problems rather than take anti-depressants forever.

We are constantly seeking a magic pill, the fountain of youth, an instant fix. We want it easy and now, and sometimes we don't look at the cost. It becomes the poisoned apple in *SnowWhite*, which promised eternal joy and delivered the kiss of death. It is time to start working on the root of the problem rather than looking for a quick fix to cover the symptom and add one more brick to the wall of disease.

You need to know how the medications, vitamins, and other supplements and chemicals affect your system. Our liver is in charge of filtering toxins. For the liver, there are only two categories of substances: food or toxin. Everything we ingest that is not real food is a toxin, and the liver has to work hard to dispose of it. Toxins are converted into a pseudo-estrogen as part of the mechanism of neutralizing and disposing of them. So each chemical we put into our bodies, from a drug to a preservative to an additive, affects the estrogen-progesterone balance. If you have been on a low-calorie diet and still are not losing weight, this may well be the reason. It doesn't matter if you are eating 800 calories a day; if they come from a shake in a can full of colorants and chemicals, or a protein bar that has a long list of ingredients that you can't pronounce and looks like a laboratory record, or a microwave frozen food that is low-fat but loaded with preservatives, your liver looks at all of that and reads, "TOXIN." There goes your hormone balance down the drain.

Think again; the short cut that you are taking when you opt for the drug's quick fix may be the longest and most miserable path. Stop, think, talk to your doctor, and look for a more natural option, keeping balance in mind as your guiding system.

In the reign of hormones, cravings are constantly plotting. The insulin-glucagon dilemma:

Once upon a time, thousands of years ago, your Paleolithic ancestors lived a life that was quite different from your modern life. According to Loren Cordain in *The Paleo Diet,* they were hunter-gatherers, which means they only ate what nature produced in its pure, unprocessed form—meat from the animals they hunted, fish, wild fruits, and vegetables. That's it. There was no dairy after breast-feeding (domesticated animals like cows were not in the picture). There were no grains (agriculture had not been invented). And, of course, there were no muffins, doughnuts, canned soups, or packaged chips. Sugar was very rare, limited to finding wild honey and the willingness to deal with the bees. Often they had to walk long distances to find food (no McDonald's around the corner). Even the composition of the meat and vegetables they ate was different. The animals fed naturally, so the meat was leaner and the vegetables were fresh, full of living enzymes and phytonutrients, and very high in fiber.

Now let's take a look at the modern diet. After the agricultural revolution, man started cultivating grains and growing cattle. We began to consume large amounts of grains (more refined as time passed) and dairy products, which was unheard of five hundred generations ago. We then created the food industry and started packaging and adding preservatives, chemicals, and artificial fats to lengthen shelf life and make food cheaper and, thus, more profitable. The result has been degenerative diseases, obesity, insulin resistance, epidemic levels of diabetes. We are just not wired or designed for this kind of diet.

A typical American consumes 150 pounds of sugar per year. He starts the day with some packaged cereal and milk, coffee, and maybe some orange juice. For lunch, he has a sandwich made with white bread and some packaged cold cuts (filled with preservatives and salt so they can last for long periods of time). The he has more coffee in the afternoon and some pastries, cookies, or candy, followed later by some pretzels (after all, they are fat free, so they must be good, right?). Dinner may be a Caesar salad loaded with bottled dressing and croutons, a steak with corn and potatoes, or chicken and rice (lots of rice), or just pizza or pasta. Oh, and some ice cream or cookies later while watching TV. That sounds pretty normal, doesn't it. Well…the truth is, it's not. At least not for our physiological constitution, which has not changed that much from our Paleolithic times.

Our brains and bodies are wired in pretty much the same fashion. We are still ruled by the balance (or imbalance) of our hormones. According to Jonny Bowden, in *Living the Low-Carb Life,* we have a "fat saving hormone" called insulin, and a "fat spending hormone," called glucagon. Insulin is in charge of communicating with our cells to open up and store sugar (that has been transformed into fat for storage) to protect our brains from an excess of sugar in the blood stream. Glucagon, on the contrary, is in charge of taking stored fat to be converted back to glucose for use as energy. When we are constantly putting sugar in our body, whether in the form of refined sugar or fast acting carbohydrates like bread, cereal, rice, potatoes, pasta, or fruit juices, the pancreas must produce very high amounts of insulin to try to normalize things and protect the brain from an excess of blood sugar. Then the muscle cells stop listening to insulin because they are already full and refuse to allow more glucose. The glucose then is converted into triglycerides (you've probably heard of them; they are a type of fat that's one of the bad guys in the fight against heart disease). If the situation continues for long enough, the tissues may ignore insulin (insulin resistance), and/or the pancreas may become exhausted and stop producing insulin, opening the way to Type II Diabetes.

Sugar has another pretty dangerous characteristic. It is highly addictive. Richard Bernstein, in his book *The Diabetes Diet,* explains why the more sugar we consume, the more we crave, in spite of its dangerous effects. Sugar promotes the release of a "feel good" neurochemical called serotonin. After consuming refined carbohydrates or sugar, a large amount of serotonin is released, thus calming our feelings of anxiety. After a short period, when the effects wear off, we go into a "low" and desperately want that feeling back, seeking more sugar or carbohydrates. It is a very potent drug with a dangerous side effect called Syndrome X, which includes obesity, high triglycerides and cardiovascular risk, and insulin resistance. Eventually this can lead to Type II Diabetes.

The good news is that exercising (especially aerobically) releases a feel good neurochemical called "endorphins" that is responsible for feelings of pleasure. Research shows that exercise also improves insulin sensitivity, helps reduce excess weight, and improves overall health. That's a good bargain when compared to sugar, isn't it?

Refined sugar is also depleted from minerals, so it uses up our minerals to be metabolized, thus depleting our reserves. It also produces AGEs (advanced glycation end products), a kind of free radical that can damage DNA, is responsible for aging and degeneration of cells, and, thus, is linked to disease. It also sticks to proteins, forming a molecule that is too big to be filtered or absorbed by capillaries, thus originating obstructions, loss of flexibility in veins, and taxing the kidneys.

So what is the good news in all this, if there is such a thing? The good news is that research shows that a change in diet and lifestyle can quickly stop and possibly reverse this downhill pattern. Dr. Richard Bernstein and other scientists agree that certain dietary changes can greatly improve our insulin sensitivity and reduce cardiovascular risk, as well as improve overall health. Again, it seems that the magic pill is nothing but education and common sense.

Loren Cordain, PhD, author of *The Paleo Diet,* recommends the following seven keys for a healthy diet. Interestingly, these same keys work to prevent cravings:

1. Eat a higher amount of protein than the typical American diet.
2. Eat fewer carbohydrates, but lots of the good carbohydrates from fruits and vegetables, not starchy tubers and refined sugars.
3. Eat more fiber.
4. Eat more mono and polyunsaturated fats than saturated fats, balancing the amount of Omega 3s and Omega 6 fats.

5. Eat foods higher in potassium and lower in sodium.
6. Eat a diet with a net alkaline load (vegetables are alkaline; sugar is acidic).
7. Eat foods rich in plant phytochemicals, vitamins, minerals, and antioxidants (fresh fruits and vegetables).

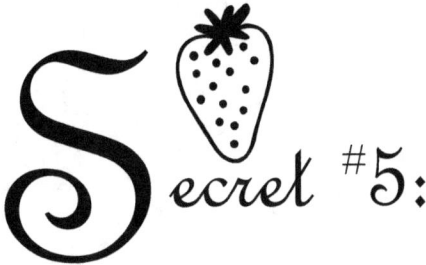

Secret #5:

Natural vs. processed

Now that you understand how your liver "thinks" you can realize why eating natural foods is so important to being healthy and fit. This section is meant to help you make wiser choices, and for that, we need your grandmother. How do you know what "food" is? Imagine going to the supermarket with your grandmother, or even better, your great grandmother. What would she buy? What would she recognize as food? She would probably skip the center isles because she would have no idea what all those packages and boxes and bags were for. She would go around the perimeter of the supermarket, and fill her shopping cart with vegetables, fruits, meat, chicken and fish, eggs, butter (the real one, not the laboratory made margarine or can't believes), olive oil, and nuts. She wouldn't get dairy because in her time, the milkman would bring to her door a container with fresh unprocessed, non-pasteurized milk from cows that ate grass and never took hormones or antibiotics, and she wouldn't buy bread because she would get it from the local baker, freshly made every day, with no sugar or preservatives.

From the earth

The more you think like her, the safer you are. Stay away from anything that has ingredients you can't pronounce. What doesn't sound like food, probably isn't. If you want to start shedding the extra pounds and stay slim and fit forever, this is a small price to pay. Instead of filling your cart with beautifully wrapped toxins, make sure you buy the following:
Cruciferous vegetables
Leafy green vegetables
Onions
Garlic
Leeks
Bitter vegetables like artichokes, celery or asparagus
Colorful vegetables like peppers, carrots, beets
Fruits

Colorful vegetables contains cancer fighting agents, colon cleansing fiber, fountain of youth anti-oxidants, liver cleansing aids, and immune system boosters. Garlic has been used for thousands of years as an anti-bacterial before antibiotics were invented. It also reduces blood pressure and cholesterol. The sulphur in onions, leeks, and garlic as well as the bitter vegetables helps the liver significantly. That is why Italians used to add garlic to everything and took a bitter drink (aperitif) with meals. A cup of broccoli or spinach contains as much calcium as a glass of milk, without the pus. I know, pfuaj!!! Did you know that the FDA ruled that up to a certain amount of pus in milk is acceptable? I don't know about you...but I don't want any amount of pus in my food, so I'll stick to my broccoli.

Apples and pears are high in pectin, a kind of fiber known for lowering cholesterol and swiping excess hormones from our body. Berries are high in antioxidants. Citrus fruits are high in vitamin C, and lemons especially are great for the liver. A cup of hot water and the juice of a fresh lemon first thing in the morning help avoid a fatty liver and keeps bile fluid, so it can better carry away toxins. All fruits are high in water, and contain beauty giving phytonutrients. They are packed with living enzymes that are needed to break down foods and assimilate them. Papaya and pineapple are so high in enzymes that they are the base of commercial meat tenderizers. "We are not what we eat, but rather what we digest, assimilate, and eliminate," says Tom Anstett, expert in Naturopathy. When we are healthy kids, we have an amazing ability to digest everything. It is very rare to hear a young child complain of being bloated, or having heartburn or constipation. Our bodies produce digestive enzymes naturally, and we also get them from fresh live fruits and vegetables. But as we grow older, sometime by our 30s, our natural production of digestive enzymes begins to decline. This is further complicated by the poor quality of the food we consume. Even when we eat a lot of vegetables and fruit, the quality is not what it used to be. Produce nowadays is picked before its ripe, stays in warehouses sometimes for weeks, then travels long distances in trucks until it gets to the supermarket. We then keep it for several days in the refrigerator until we consume it. These vegetables and fruits are far from being "alive," and they have lost a great deal of their enzymes.

Frozen fruit and vegetables sometimes are higher in nutrients than the so called fresh fruits and vegetables. They are flash frozen as soon as they are picked. Just make sure the only ingredient listed is the vegetable or fruit. Stay away from the ones with sauces, added syrups, sugars, or preservatives. None of these are necessary or add anything of value; on the contrary, they are most probably dangerous. The only ingredient in the bag must be the fruit or vegetable.

Most of us don't eat fresh locally organic or naturally grown food, so we are probably lacking enzymes and thus have poor digestion, assimilation and elimination, the three fairies of good health. We may be taking supplements and vitamins. But, what good is it if it goes out as it came in?

If you suffer from any symptom of poor digestion, assimilation, or elimination like feeling bloated or heavy after meals, constipation, heartburn, coated tongue, bad breath, or mild headaches after eating fats, you may benefit from increasing your digestive enzymes, whether it is by incorporating more fresh locally grown fruit, or by taking a good quality enzyme supplement. Just make sure to take only enzymes made of plants. Plant enzymes mimic the natural enzymes found in fresh vegetables and fruits. It is pretty much what we would get when eating better quality food. Enzymes made from animal sources like ox bile and others might contain toxins stored by those animals, and could interfere with our own production of enzymes, making the situation worse in the long run. And we want to run long, don't we?

Protein

The protein found in eggs, meat, fish, and poultry is also an important component in a healthy diet. Protein is essential for building and repairing tissues. It also helps burn fat, keep our blood sugar stable and our hunger in check in between meals. Lack of protein produces water retention and the dreaded cellulite. We have been instilled a fear of eating meat, which has been accused of causing heart disease. However, most nutrition and health scientists now agree that sugar and bad quality carbohydrates are more responsible for cardiovascular disease than meat. After being terrorized by the medical community for over a decade about the dangers of saturated fats from meat or butter, and following the prescribed fat-free diets, our risk of heart disease, diabetes, and obesity tripled. A decade ago, a breakfast consisting of a bagel with margarine, jam, and orange juice was prescribed as healthy. Why? It was fat free. Now we know the devastating effects of the blood sugar spike and insulin rush produced by the refined flour in the bagel and the sugar in the orange juice, as well as the poisonous trans-fats in margarine. Should we change that breakfast to a whole grain like oats or a sprouted grain bread like Ezekiel with real butter and a whole orange, the picture changes. When you eat an orange, the fiber slows down the absorption of sugar as opposed to drinking the juice that produces a fast shocking release. The fiber, minerals, and vitamins in the sprouted grain allow a slow and steady absorption and avoid the sugar spike, and the real butter has nutrients like Vitamin D that the body recognizes and uses.

Now, going back to meat…the problem with it is not the meat itself; it is the kind of meat you chose and what you eat with it. When you eat meat from grass fed animals that are free of hormones and antibiotics, and accompany that with a large amount of vegetables, your body is getting well-needed protein, and the vegetables allow you to digest it and carry the waste out of your body in a timely manner. When, instead, you eat regular commercial meat with potatoes, this is what you are getting: The cows from which that meat comes have been fed corn. Because nature designed their digestive system to eat grass and not corn, they get sick. So they are given tremendous amounts of antibiotics, as well as hormones to speed up the time to sell and slaughter them. Think about it, if the hormones fatten up the cows, what do you think they will do to you? On top of this, you are eating the meat without the vegetables so there are no enzymes to break down and fiber to carry out the waste. The meat will stay on your digestive track for a long, long time, and guess what happens when meat sits for long? You guessed, it putrefies. So as you can see, the problem is not eating meat, but rather eating the wrong kind of meat with the wrong side dish. The same goes for chicken. Why would you want to eat a chicken that, instead of taking the normal four months to grow, is grown in four weeks by receiving hormones? It costs a little more, but getting meat and chicken that is free of hormones and antibiotics is worth it, at least if you want to be slim and live a long time. Many well-known medical doctors and authors now agree that eating the right kind of meat is not nearly as dangerous as eating refined carbohydrates.

Eggs are another victim of bad press. They have been accused of increasing cholesterol, although the lecithin in the yolk actually helps the bile be more fluid, and plenty of research now shows that they have no impact on our cholesterol production. They also contain sulphur, which cleanses the liver and provides protein. Besides, cholesterol is nothing other than an attempt of our bodies to repair damage caused by inflammation. Think about this: A street has potholes and the road authorities send a team to put a new layer of asphalt to cover the holes and level it, so that traffic can flow without bumps. Cholesterol would be like the asphalt in our arteries: when inflammation causes bumps in the lining of our arteries, our body sends an alert and we produce cholesterol and deposit it there to level the lining and allow blood to flow smoothly. If this process repeats over and over, the arteries become narrower and the flow becomes constricted. For a long time, we have confused the attempt to repair the problem with the cause of the problem. Cholesterol is the attempt to repair; the cause of the problem is inflammation. Some current research shows that there is actually no correlation between cholesterol and heart disease. Yep...you read right. And in spite of these conclusive studies, drug companies still push the sale of cholesterol medications that ruin the liver. Why kill the messenger instead of resolving the problem? Inflammation is what causes the lining of the arteries to be rough and uneven and that, in turn, triggers cholesterol. What causes inflammation? Sugar, my dear. Have you ever cooked sugar in a pot on the stove to make caramel? Remember that sticky brown substance that forms? The same happens in your body. Sugars (and refined carbohydrates that turn into sugar) attach to proteins forming that sticky brown stuff that deposits on the arteries, making the lining rough and inflamed. That is what needs to be prevented or corrected. We need to fight the right battle. The enemy is refined sugar, not meat or eggs. If you chose not to eat meat for humanitarian or philosophical reasons, I understand. I would even agree if you are concerned about uric acid or other conditions like cancer or degenerative diseases and decide to go vegetarian. But even in that case, refined sugar is still the worst enemy. There is no point in being a vegetarian for health reasons and then eating candy, cookies, and pizza. Our ancestors have lived thousands of years eating meat from grass fed animals and plenty of vegetables before we discovered sugar and cultivated grains, so that tells us something.

Another great source of protein and nutrients, fish, used to be the cleanest and best form of animal protein…until we polluted the oceans and rivers. Nice job we did—there are all sort of toxic chemicals in what used to be our best source of food. Tuna fish is so contaminated with heavy metals that California is trying to ban its sale, and currently requires a disclaimer about its danger to pregnant women. PCVs, mercury, and who knows how many more toxic substances lurk in our previously pristine waters. However, even in this state of things, fish is still a good option when you chose the right kind. Wild Alaskan salmon, mahi, and sardines, for example, are fairly safe choices. Swordfish and tuna absorb more contaminants into their system. The smaller the fish, the less pollution it absorbs.

If you want a quick easy way to check your levels of mercury, have someone look at the back of your tongue. If you have blue branches, it is a sign of heavy metal accumulation—time to give up tuna completely and doing a good detox. The little sardine is a great choice because it is much cleaner and contains high amounts of Omega 3s (a blessing for our brains and cardiovascular system and a great warrior against inflammation). Just be careful if you have gout, since it's one of the foods in the "no" list. Fish is much easier to digest than meat or even chicken and, thus, stays less time in the digestive track, reducing the chances of releasing toxins or putrefaction. Many people chose to be "fisheterian" as an intermediate option between vegetarian and meat eaters.

Whatever you chose to do, do it for the right reasons and based on truthful information and research. Do not be fooled into thinking that eating boxed cereal is better than a good old grass fed steak.

A non-animal source of protein comes from nuts and seeds. Nuts and seeds are a blessing from nature. They contain calcium, protein, magnesium, and Omega 3s. They are a highly concentrated source of energy, so a little goes a long way (which means don't go overboard!). The trick is to eat them unsalted and raw, because when you toast them, the heat turns the good fats into bad ones. Something like what happens with olive oil, it is great on salads, but not when it's fried. The exception to this raw rule is peanuts and cashews, they tend to develop a kind of mold that is toxic; roasting or toasting reduces that risk.

A handful of raw walnuts or almonds is all you need to receive this health benefits and avoid packing on too many calories. So don't eat them from the jar or bag, just take a handful, close it and put it away before you start eating more. Since raw nuts have a great combination of good fats and protein, they activate a hormone called leptin, the "satiety hormone," that sends a message to your brain that you are full. Leptin is not activated by carbohydrates or sugars, and that is the reason why you can binge on cookies or chips so easily, your brain never gets the satiety signal and you can go on until you literally feel sick.

Raw nuts are a great snack in between meals because they won't make our blood sugar spike or trigger insulin, and they will keep us satisfied until the next meal. If you want to make them even easier to digest, you can soak them. Soaking them also destroys the phytates, a substance that inhibits the absorption of calcium. Don't be afraid of losing the crunchiness because even when you soak them for a few hours or overnight, nuts will still be crunchy and taste great.

Legumes and whole grains are wonderful and beneficial protein and fiber source. All beans are high in protein and fiber, so they are a wonderful tool for maintaining a healthy and sexy weight. Protein keeps you satisfied, and fiber helps you carry waste and toxins out of your system. On top of that, when you combine beans with whole grains, you get a complete protein, much like what you would get eating an animal food. This combination provides all the essential amino acids, with no fat and no toxins. Studies show that people who eat beans regularly lose weight faster. Worried about the gas? Start easy, with a small amount, and let your body adjust to consuming beans. Then increase slowly over a couple of weeks. If you use canned beans rinse them well in a strainer until all the foamy stuff washes away. If you cook them at home, add some sea vegetables like dulse, nori, or kelp to the water.

Grains like quinoa, millet, amaranth, and brown rice don't contain gluten, and so they won't produce inflammation of the gut. Try to avoid wheat even if you do not suffer from celiac disease or a wheat allergy. Most people suffer from a sub-clinical reaction that is not strong enough to be detected or noticed immediately, but is still there, going under the radar, unnoticed but permanently irritating the intestine.

Stay away from commercially packed so called whole grain bread. Most brands contain refined flour and just a small amount of whole grain so they can call it so, and have added preservatives and caramel coloring, which is toxic. You can now find sprouted grain breads at the supermarket in the frozen foods section. When grains are sprouted instead of refined, milled and processed, they retain minerals and enzymes and are very nutritious.

Don't believe in health claims from boxed or packaged foods. There are little or no laws as to what food manufacturers can claim in the package, and remember that their only aim is to sell that product. Nobody needs crackers or cookies or packed cereals and they don't help you achieve your ideal weight—nor do they provide nutrition.

An apple, or a celery stick, does not carry any health claim written on it and they are truly healthy and nutritious. If a food carries a health claim, it means it is processed and packaged and most probably, it is a non-food. Stay simple; eat natural, real food. Stick to real quinoa or brown rice in moderate amounts rather than "quinoa bread sticks" or "cheddar flavored rice cakes."

Oils, spices, and condiments

Not all fats are created equal, and discrimination is a good quality when it comes to fats. Essential fatty acids are, as their name establishes, essential for blood vessels and nerves, and to keep the skin and other tissues supple, lubricated, and young. The ratio between Omega 3 and Omega 6 essential fatty acids determines the flexibility of cell membranes, so all chemical communication between our organs and systems depends on this balance. Our primitive ancestors, who ate naturally, consumed far more Omega 3 than Omega 6 fats. The ratio in their diet was one to one. In the modern American diet, on the contrary, the ratio is between ten to one and twenty to one. That means Americans consume up to twenty times more Omega 6 than needed. Most of the oils consumed here contain Omega 6—soybean oil, canola oil, corn oil. By choosing olive, flaxseed, chia seed, or pumpkin seed oil instead, we are helping to correct this imbalance. If we could chose salmon instead of chicken and walnuts instead of peanuts more often, we would be helping this balance as well.

One important caution about oil is that when we use them raw, like in salads or on top of vegetables after cooking them, they provide all those health benefits, but when we heat them, not only we destroy the benefits, but we also transform them into a toxic substance. Flaxseed oil is especially susceptible to heat, so please never cook with it. It needs to be refrigerated. Olive oil is also sensitive to heat. Contrary to common belief, coconut oil has many health benefits and resists high temperatures, so is one of the few oils suitable for sautéing or cooking. It is also an amazing skin moisturizer, and leaves a tropical vacation smell on your skin that lifts the mood at the same time.

One of the reasons why the Mediterranean diet is considered so healthy is its preference for olive oil. At least 2 tablespoons a day are necessary for lubrication of the intestines and proper elimination. And if you suffer from dry eyes, consuming flax seed or chia seed oil over time eliminates the problem, and in my experience, they are more effective than using eye drops, which only offer temporary relief.

While the right oil is good for cooking, one easy step you can take for the sake of your health and your waistline is to either steam or water sauté instead of stir-frying. Just use some broth to cook your vegetables, and only after you remove them from heat, add some olive oil for a delicious flavor.

Don't forget to spice up your life either. Spices contain a treasure of phytochemicals with medicinal and health giving properties. Our culture is so used to relying on salt to give taste to our food that we have polluted our taste buds and everything tastes the same. Spices add variety and sophistication. They help digestion and raise our metabolism. They also have many therapeutic uses, so before you go to the pharmacy…check your kitchen spice shelf.

Most herbal spices prevent and relieve gas and help digestion. Some are also good for nervousness, spasms, and coldness. They can be used to treat conditions like diarrhea, infections, headaches, and bleeding. They are a safe and natural alternative to synthetic drugs. They can be considered "crisis medicine," treating the first acute stages of disease. Play with them, use them often in your cooking, and take advantage of the healing properties of these natural wonders. My favorite trio is turmeric, ginger, and cayenne. Turmeric is an amazingly powerful natural anti-inflammatory, and as you already know by now, inflammation is the real cause of many diseases, including cardiovascular problems. Ginger is a natural anti-bacterial—kind of an internal antiseptic. Cayenne raises your metabolism with its thermogenic properties and burns waste matter in your system. In India, ayurvedic medicine considers that the cause of any disease is an accumulation of "ama," or toxins and waste material. Cayenne is recommended to get rid of ama. The trick is moderation, since this is one of the hot spices. A little is enough to receive the benefits, and unless it is cooked, most people tolerate it well. Check with your doctor if you suffer from ulcers, ulcerative

colitis, or IBS, although some naturopathic doctors have success-
fully used it uncooked even in that case.

Here's a list of common spices and their use:

Anise: It breaks up mucus and helps dry coughs. Let three teaspoons
of crushed seeds steep for twenty minutes in a cup of boiling water.
Add honey to taste.

Basil: Use for a fever. Make tea with one ounce of basil leaves to
one pint of simmering water twenty minutes. Add three powdered
black peppercorns per cup.

Bay: Add to beans and soups to prevent gas and indigestion.

Black pepper: It is an excellent first aid remedy for the first sign
of most diseases. One eighth teaspoon powder mixed with honey
helps with cold, mucous diseases and sore throats. At the acute
stage, it can be taken three times a day.

Caraway: It is good for indigestion, colic, and gas. Steep an ounce
of crushed seeds in a pint of boiling water for twenty minutes. Take
two tablespoons at a time until relief is obtained.

Cayenne: Used as a stimulant, astringent, carminative, and antispasmodic, it is a superior crisis remedy and for first aid for most
conditions. When uncooked, cayenne is not irritating. For arthri-
tis, a little cayenne can be rubbed over the inflamed joint and
wrapped with a flannel overnight. The pain is usually gone by the
morning.

Cinnamon: Simmered in milk with a little honey, it helps indigestion, gas, and diarrhea. It is also very helpful in regulating blood
sugar levels.

Cumin: It is one of the best spices to prevent gas. Add it to beans and hard to digest foods.

Fennel: It can be used as an antispasmodic, carminative, diuretic, expectorant, and stimulant. Steeping one teaspoon of crushed seeds in a cup of boiling water for twenty minutes helps relieve gas and expel mucus.

Fenugreek: It is good to relieve congestion and eliminate mucus, and useful for ulcers and inflamed conditions of stomach and intestines. One ounce of crushed seeds and seven crushed black peppercorns in a pint of water are used to make a decoction.

Garlic: This world renowned cure-all remedy is used as expectorant, an antibiotic, to fight parasites and infections, to regulate blood pressure, and more. For healing effects, it should not be boiled or cooked. Fresh juice is the best form.

Ginger: It is excellent for indigestion, cramps, and nausea (don't forget it when going on a cruise!). Simmer one ounce of fresh ginger in a pint of water for ten minutes. With honey and lemon, it is great for colds and flu. Add it to meat dishes to help the intestines detoxify the meat.

Rosemary: It is a natural substitute for aspirin. Steep a half ounce in a pint of boiled water for ten minutes.

Thyme: It is good as a parasiticide for intestinal worms, and good for bronchitis and laryngitis. Steep an ounce in one pint of boiling water, strain, and sweeten with honey.

Turmeric: This great anti-inflammatory is also good as a blood purifier and to reduce fevers and nosebleed. A teaspoon of turmeric and one teaspoon of almond oil in a cup of warm milk twice a day is an ayurvedic remedy for cramps.

Oregano: It has anti-fungal and anti-parasite properties and works on an emotional level to address fears.

Cilantro: It helps destroy bacteria like e-coli.

Be creative; start using herbs and spices rather than salt. You will not only correct the potassium-salt imbalance, but also receive innumerable benefits and nutrients.

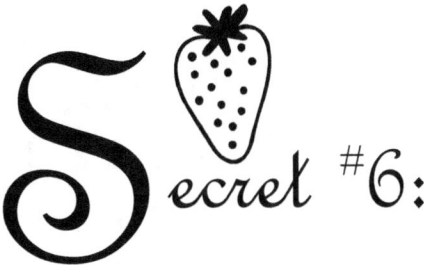

Secret #6:

Be like the ameba, stay
away from what's bad

The ameba is a tiny little microscopic unicellular organism. You've probably seen it in the school lab under a microscope in a drop of water from a street puddle. And you probably never thought too much about it either. You'd better start, because the ameba teaches us something that we, with all our millions of brain cells, don't remember: "Move toward what is good for you, and move away from what is bad for you." That simple, and the simple tiny ameba knows how to do this.

Translated into our more complicated life and weight goals, we need to move toward the foods that keep us healthy and slim, and stay away from the saboteurs. In this chapter, we will discuss all the common saboteurs so that we can, like the ameba, avoid them.

The first saboteur is refined sugar: Refined sugar activates the release of insulin, which, as you remember from Secret #4, is the fat saving hormone. A good rule is to save your money and spend your fat. Refined sugar is also the evil behind silent or sub-clinical inflammation, cardiovascular disease, yeast infections, candida and fungus, cravings, mood swings, and weight gain. Cancer cells thrive on sugar, and bacteria reproduces in sugar. It causes many other conditions we don't want.

I am a big fan of linguistics, and am always amazed at the effect that the words we chose have on our mood and behavior. I was once talking with a client that came for weight management. She was telling me about an argument with her husband (that led her to finish the Oreo cookies later that night), and described his position saying, "That's bullshit!." I immediately thought how curious it is that we use the excrement of an animal to represent something we disagree with because we think is fake or false. Bull shit (or cow shit) happens to be a truthful organic fertilizer that serves an important purpose. It is natural and honest. It does not mislead us; its smell and appearance make the fact that it is not something edible very obvious. Sugar, in contrast, serves absolutely no positive purpose or function. (Please note I am not talking about blood sugar or the kind of sugar that fuels our brain, but about the refined white powder that is slowly but surely killing us.) It tricks us into thinking it's great through an attractive taste and appearance. It makes us addicted to it by producing a spike of fake energy and pleasure while in reality it is the beginning of the crash. It produces candida and feeds bacteria, which will reproduce and overpower our immune system—which by the way becomes suppressed for several hours every time we consume refined sugar. It turns into a sticky brownish substance that binds to proteins and clogs our arteries. Since the refinement process has depleted white sugar from minerals, it uses our mineral reserve to be metabolized. It makes our bodies acidic, so that in order to restore pH balance, we consume our calcium, and if there is not enough calcium around, we pull it from our bones, which, over time, leads to osteoporosis. It makes us fat and weak.

So, who is here the impostor, the fake one, the perpetrator? Bull shit or sugar? I shared my thoughts about this with my client and suggested that from now on, every time she wants to refer to something false, with no value, or upsetting, she uses the word "sugar" instead of "bullshit." By doing that, her mind will create a negative association with sugar that by repetition will become a habit and change her perception of sugar. She looked at me as if I was crazy but promised to give it a shot.

The following session she came in smiling. She couldn't stop laughing when telling me about her family and friend's face every time someone said something stupid and she screamed, "that's sugar!." It worked for her' she progressively cut down on sugar as she kept doing this. Suddenly, cookies, sodas, and deserts lost their pull and power over her. As she became free from her sugar addiction and lost weight, she regained not only her figure, but also her good mood. Why not give it a shot? The next time you are watching the news and hear nonsense, or someone tries to trick you, forcefully say, "that's sugar" and you may be pleasantly surprised with the change it brings.

Artificial sweeteners are no better. Your brain does not distinguish between real or artificial sugar, so every time you eat or drink a "diet" product artificially sweetened, it sends a signal to the pancreas to secrete insulin. But insulin does not find any sugar to attach to, so it sends back a signal to the brain to make you crave sugars or carbohydrates. Have you noticed that every time you drink diet sodas you get hungry or have cravings soon after? Studies show that people who drink water lose much more weight than those drinking diet sodas—all other factors being equal. Aspartame has been linked to Alzheimer's and Splenda to stomach problems. Stay away from them!

The next saboteur is gluten and refined flour. Refined flour has been stripped from every benefit a grain might have—minerals and fiber—and it is a non food that quickly turns into sugar after we eat it, so all that we discussed before about sugar applies here as well. Gluten is found in wheat and other grains like barley and rye. In people with celiac disease, it causes an allergic reaction that produces diarrhea and peels away the cilia, those little hairs in the gut through which nutrients are absorbed. In some cases it can be severe enough to require hospitalization. Although very few people have celiac disease, most of us have a sub-clinical reaction to gluten. This means we don't get the full-blown allergic reaction, but rather a minor but consistent inflammation in the gut that over time takes a toll in our health, causing conditions like indigestion, weight gain, bloating, gas, skin reactions, asthma, and other allergic reactions that most doctors would never think of linking to gluten. But the truth is that, in many cases, when people suffering from these disorders are put on a gluten free diet, their condition dramatically improves. Gluten is not a healthy substance for any of us and, unfortunately, it is not only used in breads, pastries, and crackers, which we don't need anyways, but also in salad dressings, sauces, cold cuts, and most processed foods. Remember the ameba, stay away from them! Grains like quinoa, amaranth, brown rice, and millet are gluten free.

Now let's talk about two saboteur that have managed to convince us that they actually have some benefits: caffeine and alcohol. Coffee raises our cortisol by 300 percent to 400 percent. And remember what cortisol does? It makes you ravenously hungry for fatty and highly caloric foods, and stores those calories as fat in your waistline and belly area. It also produces a fake spike in energy followed by a crash. Since it creates a very acidic pH, it forces our body to pull calcium from our bones in order to correct the alkaline-acid balance. It is also dehydrating. Three cups of coffee per day can result in a 45-mg calcium loss. Coffee lovers protest saying that it has anti-oxidants, but after reading this, doesn't it make sense to get your anti-oxidants from vegetables and fruits? Remember that you are getting much more caffeine than you think, not just in coffee but also in sodas, chocolate, and medications like Exedrin and many others sold over the counter.

We've all heard that a glass of wine is good for the heart. This is because it contains reservatrol, a powerful anti-oxidant, which we can easily get by eating some grapes instead. Although it may be true that a glass of wine has some health benefits, it is also true that it puts a strain on the liver—and, often, that one glass quickly turns into two or three. Alcohol turns into sugar, and it lowers our ability to control our impulses. After a glass or two of alcohol, it becomes very easy to forget your weight goal and your decision to be fit, and without even noticing, eat the bread, chips and pretzels, or dessert. Although some people believe alcohol is relaxing and it helps them sleep or have better sex, the truth is that research shows it negatively affects the quality of both sleep and sex.

Two other things to avoid are fried foods and trans fats. Trans fats are created when vegetable oils are hydrogenated, producing a solid and semi solid fat commonly used in commercial baked goods, processed foods, and at fast food restaurants. Trans fats make food manufacturers happy by providing a longer shelf life; but they interfere with our liver's ability to burn fat and detoxify, and they thicken bile. Margarine, hydrogenated oils, and shortening are all trans fats and if we follow the ameba's advise, we'll stay away from them. Fried foods produce toxins, accelerated metabolic aging, and

AGEs (advanced glycation end products), which not only are linked to cancer, but are the cause of aging and degenerative diseases.

Instead of frying and using fats, many of us choose the healthier form of cooking, grilling. But is grilling really healthy? According to Dr. Steven Joyal, M.D., from Dartmouth, grilling meat, poultry, or fish is far from being healthy. When meat is subjected to dry heat of more than 250 degrees, it produces glycotoxins. The Maillard reaction is the scientific name for what we normally call browning. That crispy browning is not innocent, it means that glycation, or glycotoxins, have formed. Glycotoxins accelerate the aging process, and who wants to age faster? This is not just about getting wrinkles; the aging acceleration also involves degenerative processes that may cause cancer, Alzheimer's, and other conditions we'd better avoid. The solution? Cook meat, fish, or poultry with liquid. You can make them in a stew, or cook them in broth and white wine. This method is delicious, keeps the moisture, and, most important, avoids glycotoxins. Steaming works well too, especially with fish. Or use a crock pot; it uses very low heat over long periods of time, so you can prepare it in the morning, and when you come home from work, dinner is ready and warm.

Another step you can take to counteract the effect of glyco-toxins is to eat apples, onions, tea, and chocolate (yes, you have yet another good excuse!). They are all rich in flavonoids or quercetin, two heroes in the battle against cell degeneration and free radicals.

Another product thought to be better than it is for us is dairy. Humans are the only species that, after being breastfed by our mothers, continue breast feeding from other animals. It is so unnatural that most adults lose the ability to produce an enzyme necessary to digest lactose and get unpleasant reactions like digestive problems, diarrhea, respiratory problems, excess mucus, congestion, and allergies. To make matters worse, the milk we drink nowadays has been pasteurized, a process that changes the molecules, making it even more difficult to digest. Our cows are fed corn, which makes them sick, and over milked, which produces infections in their nipples, which causes the pus I talked about earlier. I don't know about you, but I don't want any amount of pus in my food. In England there was a campaign mocking our milk consumption that showed a skinny model with a milk mustache that read "Got pus?"

Once you then add the hormones and antibiotics, it is not a pretty substance to ingest. But even in the case of organic milk, it is still linked to the allergic reactions mentioned above. We don't need milk to get calcium. Broccoli, leafy greens, and almonds are all a great sources of calcium. By eating much more vegetables than animal products, our bodies will maintain the acid-alkaline optimal balance and we won't need to pull calcium from our bones to balance the excess acidity.

Cheese is also high in sodium and fat. The only exception is natural plain yogurt or kefir, because the good bacteria in them has pre-digested the lactose, making it easy on us and helping our intestinal flora balance with its probiotics. If you still insist on drinking milk, go for goat's milk, it is much easier on your system.

Lastly, stay away from processed foods as much as you can. Go back to Secret #5 and read it again every time you are tempted to go for the apparently easy processed non-food. The chemicals, additives, colorants, preservatives, and high fructose corn syrup are dangerous enemies diligently plotting against your liver and, thus, your waistline. Remember, anything that your body doesn't recognize as food is a toxin; and once we overpass our capacity to get rid of toxins, we start storing them in fat—the more toxins, the more fat.

And now let's talk about another kind of saboteur. We all have "friends" and relatives that get very uncomfortable when we decide to eat healthy, lose weight, and look gorgeous. They are the ones who say, "What is one slice of cake going to do?" or "I cooked it especially for you," or "Life is too short, enjoy and don't worry about calories." You have two choices here: stay away from them or learn to become assertive and defend your decision to live better and be slim. They are scared about your decision because you are reminding them of the fact that they are ruining their health, and maybe that they also need to lose weight. They are scared about losing you as a partner in crime. They are scared because your decision shakes their world and they don't want to think about the damage they are doing to themselves. They are scared that you will become more attractive.

I encourage you to surround yourself with friends that also care about their health and eat good food. It will make it easier for you. In some cases, this is not possible because the saboteur may be a close friend, a relative, or a spouse. Often, when the wife decides to lose weight, the husband brings her chocolates, or eats ice cream in front of her, or suddenly starts buying candy and cookies. It all comes from their fear of having their wife become the object of desire for other men, and the fear of being abandoned. If this happens to you, just make an extra effort to reassure him of your love and ask him for his help to stick to your goal. Men like to be needed. Also, learn to be assertive and polite. When someone insists on you having "just a bite of the pie," say, "I am sure it is delicious and I appreciate the time and effort you put in making it, but I am not going to have it." You can also say that you are not eating that "for health reasons." It is hard to argue with that. You will feel so good about yourself after you leave the event without betraying your goal, that the satisfaction of that will be bigger than any momentary pleasure of your taste buds.

Avoid places that trigger a memory of unhealthy eating. Why go for coffee to that French bakery that has the éclairs you used to crave? Why not go to places that have healthy options instead? Learn from the ameba, stay away from what is bad for you.

Are you sharing a fatty bond with your friends? Are you used to going for doughnuts or pizza and beer? Change it, start coming up with ideas that involve healthy food or no food at all. Why not meet for a walk? Why not share a movie or a book club or a dance class instead? You will discover that you can still have fun and share great times while winning the battle of the skinny jeans.

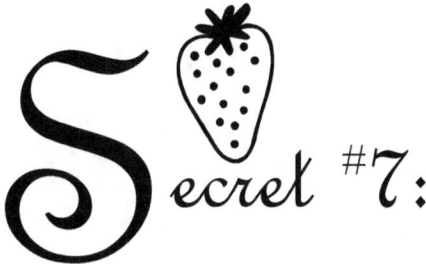

Secret #7:

Plan

"If I had 3 hours to cut down a tree,
I would spend 2 and a half sharpening the ax,"
Abraham Lincoln.

Being prepared is one of the secrets for success in any area, including achieving and maintaining your perfect weight. Let's look at some common scenarios:

1. You come home after work tired and cranky, with nothing planned for dinner. You open the pretzel jar and start snacking on that while you call for pizza.

2. You have a busy day at the office and lunch time comes with no plan; you eat some of the bagels in the coffee room, or order some fast food.

3. You go to a birthday party with no plan; you find yourself joining the "eat cake" team.

4. You wake up late and have to rush out; you quickly grab a breakfast bar or cookies on your way out.

5. You have a fight with your boyfriend and eat a whole ice cream container full of your favorite flavor.

What do all these scenarios have in common? In all of them, you have set yourself up for failure by not having a plan. Let's see how all these falling-off-the-wagon scenarios could have been avoided by good planning:

1. You come home from work tired and cranky, but this time you have hummus and celery sticks already washed and cut in the refrigerator. You also have some frozen vegetables and quinoa pasta so you can put together a delicious and healthy pasta primavera in just ten minutes, less than what the pizza takes to arrive!

2. You have a busy day at the office; lunch time comes and you already have a sandwich you brought from home made with Ezekiel sprouted bread, avocado, turkey, lettuce, and tomato. Or you open the first drawer in your desk and have menus and phone numbers for healthy restaurants that deliver, so you order a big nice salad with salmon.

3. You go to a birthday party, and you take a beautiful vegetable platter to share and inspire others to join the "I care about me" team. You also eat some raw nuts before you leave so you are not starving.

4. You wake up late and have to rush, so you grab a delicious crunchy apple on your way out.

5. You have a fight with your boyfriend, so you sit quietly and write in your journal about the need that each of you was trying to communicate and couldn't. Or you call a friend that knows how to listen and talk your frustration out.

What is the common thread in all of the second option behaviors? You had a plan. You can't expect to choose celery and hummus if you only have pretzels at home. You need to make a list every week, go food shopping and buy only (and I mean only) what's on your list. Your refrigerator and pantry need to be packed with success foods—no saboteurs allowed!

You need to have a list of "quick fix" healthy foods for those times when you are in a rush. You need to have a plan and stick to it; but how can you stick to a plan if you don't have one to begin with? Going to a party? Make a mental list of what you are going to have; take something with you and eat something before you go. When you know beforehand what you are going to have for each meal, it is much more probable that you won't succumb to that automatic behavior that put you in trouble with your weight. You will also make sure that you are eating balanced foods. To make your life easier, you need a "success list" of at least five breakfast, lunch, snack, and dinner options, and carry that list with you wherever you go. When you are hungry, look at your list and pick one item. That way you won't be lost; your mind will be focused on finding that choice instead of overwhelmed and confused by all the destructive offers of the food industry.

Before you go to a restaurant, before you open the menu, you need to make a choice from your "success list." Only then look at the menu to find something that matches your choice. Now you have a goal, you are no longer a victim of your hormones, your company's influence, or your automatic drive. You can also tell the waiter to take away the bread, or not to bring any in the first place. Just be polite and ask your company if they agree. You'll be surprised that most people will be grateful and admire your commanding attitude. You can share a plate with your partner or friend, or ask for a takeout container to put half of your plate in before you start to eat (then close it and put it in a bag). Portions are usually at least two times bigger than what we need, and it is easy to continue eating until the plate is empty, unless you plan otherwise. Ask for dressings and sauces on the side. Restaurants tend to put three to five times more dressing than necessary, and just the dressing on that salad can have 600 calories. The same is true sauces, and they are also usually very high in salt, fat, and sugar, which make them addictive and drives you to eat more than you need. By ordering dressings and sauces on the side, you can control how much you use; just a tablespoon or two can be enough to give flavor, while keeping your choice still healthy and your calories within range. Or just ask for no dressing at all, and get olive oil and lemon for the table instead, which you can add to your salad or food and control how much you use.

As to dessert, most restaurants now carry the shot glass version of any dessert, which helps control the amount and keep the splurge within reasonable limit. Or if you are dining with at least three other people, chose one dessert for the table and share it. You may be surprised to find out that just a few teaspoons are all you really wanted.

For your food shopping list, remember to include all the "yes" foods in Chapter 5—a large variety of vegetables (frozen and fresh) of all colors, plain yogurt, sprouted Ezekiel bread, quinoa pasta, quinoa, brown rice, millet, beans, sprouts, an assortment of fruits, spices, canned and fresh salmon, sardines, turkey, hormone and antibiotic free chicken and eggs, grass fed meat, hummus, raw nuts and seeds, sea vegetables like kelp and dulse, and dried figs (for a healthy treat). When you are surrounded by healthy foods, you'll end up making healthy choices. Purge your home of anything that can sabotage your goal. Don't lie to yourself saying that you are keeping those chocolates in case you have visits; you know what will happen. Don't rationalize that you have potato chips for your husband and kids; they don't need them either. If you want to succeed, be merciless!

Talk to your spouse and kids, let them know how important this is to you, tell them you want to be healthy and look good for you and for them, and that you need their support and understanding. Your kids don't need junk food and if you care about them, you'll show them the way.

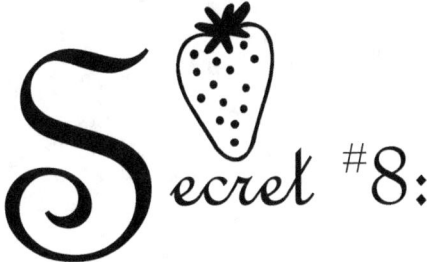

Secret #8:

Damage Control

Let's suppose you decide to go on a road trip from town "A" to town "B." The total travel time is ten hours. Three hours after leaving your hometown, "A," you get a flat tire. What do you do? Do you change it and continue toward "B" or do you go back to "A," where you started? Let's suppose you continue driving, and two hours later, the route is closed for repairs, so you need to take a detour that will signify an extra hour of driving. Do you follow the detour and continue to "B" or turn around and go back home? I can bet my retirement that you answered yes to the first questions (change the tire, take detour and continue). Maybe you decide to skip the next stop to make up for lost time, or maybe you just arrive at "B" a couple of hours later than expected; the point is, you arrive. Now please someone explain this to me. How come in the road trip, you solve the inconvenience, accept the delay and continue toward your destination, but in a journey toward the new fit you, when a challenge arises, you give up everything you achieved and go back to the starting point (or worse, further back)? Does it make any sense? Nope. But that's what you've been doing. You follow your eating plan, you start shedding the extra pounds little by little. Then you have a dinner party and although you were determined to "be a good girl," the fried spring rolls looked so good, and after a cocktail or two, you tried one, and another. Now you say to yourself "I already ruined it, I might as well enjoy and eat the bread as well, and the cake," and you eat everything you can as if it is the end of the world, the last supper. Then you go back home feeling bloated and guilty, and your mind goes round and around telling you how bad you are, what a failure you are, that you'll NEVER be thin, you have no will power, and on and on. The next morning, you step on the scale and you feel like the most worthless worm, so you continue eating crap and tell yourself you will start again on Monday. However, by that Monday you have gained all the pounds shed and some more.

What if you took the same attitude as on the road trip? What if after a minor slip like the cocktail or the spring roll you tell yourself it's a minor delay, nothing to worry about, and you go back to your map, your plan. Maybe the next day you choose even more vegetables than usual and eat lighter to make up for the night before, or maybe you just go back to your eating plan like nothing happened, knowing that it is possible you will achieve your goal a couple of days later. What's the big deal? You may be surprised to realize that by the end of the week you still lost a couple of pounds. The point here is to stop the self-deprecating thoughts, shut down that abusive inner voice that causes the feeling of guilt and worthlessness and reassure yourself. Bring the example of the road trip to your awareness; remind yourself that the inconvenience is just a detour, or a flat tire, and that you can fix it and still arrive at your destination and have the time of your life. Give up the black or white kind of thinking (i.e., either you are perfect or you are a failure). There are hundreds of shades of gray. You can be effective and still have room for mistakes.

I can also give you two more reasons why a "slip" is not a tragedy. First, a slip can be a valuable source of information to get to know yourself better and improve your plan (like the radio shows that use the info on accidents and detours to warn drivers and provide an alternative route). Journaling is a great tool to decipher your inner codes of action. In Secret #1, we spoke about using journaling to discover how your body reacts to different foods. We can add one more step here and maximize the benefits of journaling to include valuable information about what drives you to eat. When you keep a "mood and food" journal, you will start to see connections and patterns that once discovered can be avoided. To keep that kind of journal, divide the pages into four columns: time, food, situation, and mood. For example, 3:00 p.m., a muffin, right after call from boss, pressured. Or 10.30 p.m. ice cream, watching TV, lonely. This kind of information is extremely useful, almost like the GPS on the road trip. You will start to notice patterns; you will soon be able to pinpoint the triggers. This has a double benefit. On one hand, by becoming your own observer, you are stepping out of the situation and objectively witnessing (pretty much what happens in awareness meditation). Once you step out, you can think with a clear head. Second, when you understand the patterns and triggers, you can plan accordingly (I know I tend to feel lonely at night, I will make a plan with my friend X who goes to sleep late and call her if I feel that way, I will also have some nuts and some apple slices microwaved with cinnamon, lemon, and a little agave so that I have a healthy warm delicious late night snack if I feel like). I recently heard a man, who went from over 400 pounds to less than 200 pounds and has maintained it for five years, say, "It is a lack of respect toward sadness to cover it with food." Staying with your feelings, being able to really feel them, is the best you can do for yourself. "Everything that comes to the light can be healed." Don't be afraid to be overpowered by feelings. When you allow yourself to feel your sadness, frustration or anger, they will naturally and spontaneously recede. If, instead, you ignore them, repress them, deny them, or cover them with food, they will never go away, and they will find a destructive way for expression. Just acknowledge what you feel; be respectful of anything you feel. Tell yourself, "I am feeling…and that's OK." Use your food and mood journal to understand the connection between situations, relationships, mood, and food (e.g., Do you eat cookies every time you call your mom?). This practice will be something like turning on the light in a dark room. You will be amazed at the things you find, and it will be so much easier to put things in order now rather than in the dark.

Maybe you find that one of the feelings that is currently driving you to eat is anxiety. If you are anxious, come back! Racing thoughts, sweaty palms, fast beating heart, and that knot…we all know the sensation of being anxious, and it is definitely not a pleasant one. Why do we get anxious? A million people will give a million different answers, but I can summarize them all in one: Because we step out of the "now" and into the future. Anxiety is future based; it is always related to fear of an event that may or may not exist…in the future. Mark Twain said "My life has been filled with horrible events that never happened." My mother would say, "Why worry now, when you can worry tomorrow."

The bottom line is…it does not exist now, in this precise instant. That means that if you can keep your focus in the present moment, you have chased anxiety away. "Very nice," you might be saying, "but how do I do that?" The easiest way is to screen your body. Start with your feet—can you feel your feet planted on the floor? How does it feel? Move up to your legs—what sensation do you feel in your legs? Are they cold, warm, tense, relaxed, achy? What about your back? Where is there tension; where is there comfort? Can you feel the touch of your clothes? Go up in this way until you have checked in with your head, hair, face, eyes, arms, shoulders, and hands. If thoughts intrude your screening, just observe them, as if they were a bird crossing the sky, then disappearing, don't judge them, just let them be...and watch them leave.

Another option is to imagine a white screen, where every thought is a black dot. Your job is to keep the screen white. Want yet another one? Just follow your breath, without trying to change it. Pay attention to the feeling of the air passing through your nose— the temperature, the movement, the length and depth—without attempting to do anything with it other than observe. By becoming an observer, you are automatically stepping back in the "now," where anxiety has no place. As Eckart Tolle said, "Do not worry about the future, the future will take care of itself."

The second reason why a slip is not only not a tragedy, but sometimes a good thing, is that you can have planned slips that work for you. Your metabolism is ruled by a delicate hormonal monitoring system. Keep in mind that our primitive ancestors didn't have such a plentiful life. Food was scarce and the risk of dying from lack of it was high. So nature put a protection mechanism in our hormones—when the caloric intake is reduced, the metabolism (the speed at which we burn calories for energy) slows down. And we still carry that program. It takes approximately seven days for hormones to make the decision that food is scarce and signal our metabolism to slow down. That's what happens behind a plateau (I was losing weight and now all of a sudden the scale doesn't move, even though I am following my plan). So, if once a week you incorporate a planned "slip," you will avoid the slowing down of your metabolism. Please be aware that when I talk about a planned slip,

I am not referring to an endless day of junk eating. I am just talking about choosing ONE thing that normally is not part of your plan. Maybe pasta on Sundays for dinner, or pizza or a dessert once a week. Please note the presence of the word "or" and avoid substituting it for "and" to make this work for you instead of against you.

This planned "slip" will reassure your hormones that there is no scarcity of food, no danger of famine, and, thus, no need to slow down your metabolism for the next seven days, at which time you will pick another planned "slip." The extra calories of the pizza, pasta, or whatever choice you make will be more than compensated for by avoiding a slowdown of your metabolism. This strategy will also be a good practice to learn to avoid the black or white mentality. It will be an exercise in avoiding extremes (if I eat one thing out of my plan I start an all day binge), teaching you that it is possible to move a few steps away from your route without rolling down an abyss. Furthermore, it will retrain your brain out of guilt and abusive self-talk when you eat something out of the ordinary. Notice that I say "out of the ordinary" and not "forbidden." This is precisely the key point here—there is nothing forbidden, it is only a matter of how often you chose to eat certain foods. So, there is no more guilt associated with those foods any more.

Secret #9:

Know thyself. Hunger or anger?
Nurture or nourishment?

It is very easy to confuse emotions like anger, anxiety, pain, a need for love, or loneliness with hunger. And this is not your fault; it's the way nature wired us to ensure survival. Remember that primitive men were primarily hunters (agriculture was invented much, much later). So the sensation of hunger was linked to a violent drive to kill. Hunger was mixed with a feeling of irritability and anger, a way to fuel the impulse to go kill a beast, so we could eat, and then, and only then, feel relaxed. That connection between anger and hunger is still imprinted in our brains, so that when we are angry or irritable, we start feeling hungry or thinking of food.

Another example is the need for love, which is universal. When we are born, we are absolutely vulnerable. We cannot survive without our mom (or someone in her place), taking care of us and feeding us. In order to increase our chances of survival, nature came up with a creative solution: as babies, hunger and pain feel the same way. When a baby is hungry, it is in pain. That makes the baby cry and cry without stopping, until the mother provides survival through her feeding breast. That is also the reason why when babies have colic, produced by a still immature digestive system, they only stop crying when they are put to the breast again, even though what they need is to give their stomach a rest. But, as we said, they cannot differentiate between hunger and pain. Feeding also comes with loving contact; mom holds the baby in her arms providing not only nourishment but nurturing, protection, safety, and attention. That experience is stored in our subconscious memory. We carry that association between food, safety, love, and relief from pain into adulthood. How many times have you found yourself reaching for food when you feel scared, lonely or in pain? It has even turned into a movie cliché: the woman eating ice-cream after a break-up.

Although, as I said before, this is not your fault, it is your responsibility. Why? Because if you don't work at understanding and consciously changing these habits, nobody will do it for you. Once again, awareness is the answer. Every time you feel an urge to eat, you can take a moment to check inside what is truly happening. If you had a nice lunch at 12.30, and you are hungry a couple of hours later, what is the reason? Have you had a meal too rich in carbohydrates and sugar that produced a spike and crash in blood sugar levels? Or have you had a thought that made you feel angry or anxious? Are you irritable because you woke up too early and didn't sleep well? What were you thinking or doing right before you thought of food? Is your neck, shoulders, or jaw tight and tense? Do you feel a knot in your throat or chest? The way you feel in your body can give you clues. Tight and tense muscles may indicate anger and anxiety. The knot in your chest or throat could be apprehension or fear of putting something into words. Follow that lead—what is it that you resist putting into words?

You need to decide consciously if you actually have a need for food at this precise moment, because if you leave that decision to your subconscious, it will attempt to resolve every negative emotion with food. That's the default mode your subconscious mind brings built in, and what it further learned as a baby.

In biological terms, we have a primitive brain, called the amygdale, which is in charge of automatic responses and impulses. We also have a more sophisticated and developed part of the brain, called the frontal lobe, which is in charge of analytical thinking and processing. Both of them are necessary. If a piano is falling from a balcony and you are standing right underneath it, you can't afford the luxury of engaging the frontal lobe to analyze options, think about the moral ramifications, compare alternatives, and so on. You need your amygdale to quickly sense danger and drive you to jump to the side in a fraction of a second. But when you are about to reach for a muffin to placate your feeling of pressure and anxiety about a deadline at work, you need your frontal lobe to analyze and understand what is really going on, and determine that it's not food you need, but a relaxing break instead.

Whether you choose to think about it as awareness, your conscious mind you're your frontal lobe, your responsibility in this game is to reach for that part of you that is capable of taking the time to make the right choice. Here is an example of the tricky ways in which our subconscious stores and uses information.

Karen was a forty-six-year-old overweight woman. She had been overweight for as long as she could remember. She had read every diet book and tried every diet on the market for decades with no result. South Beach, Atkins, Jenny Craig, vegetarian, dissociated, low-carb, macrobiotic…you name it, she had tried it, always to end disappointed and frustrated with maybe a couple of pounds less, which quickly crept on again. I could see her struggle to hold the tears as she told me about her story. I asked Karen, "Do you want to lose weight?" She looked at me with a mix of surprise and indignation at the stupidity of the question. "Why do you think I am here?," she said. "Why do you think I have failed with all these diets and am still trying?" I explained that the fact that wanting something consciously does not mean all of your mind agrees, and proceeded to muscle test her. (In case you are unfamiliar with muscle testing, it is a technique in which you ask a question and it is the body that responds instead of the mind—by the changes in muscle strength. I love this technique because in my experience, the mind can trick you and rationalize anything and everything, but your body never lies.) So I asked her a couple of questions to familiarize her with the procedure. "Is your name Karen?," and her arm stayed strong and firm (indicating her agreement with no resistance or contradictory feelings). "Where you born in Philadelphia?," again, strong arm. "Do you want to lose weight?" Her arm went completely limp, and fell down like a rag doll. Karen was in shock. "I don't understand it," she cried, "I do want to lose weight; there is nothing I want more than that. I would give anything to achieve it." I explained that her subconscious mind obviously disagreed with that idea, and since the subconscious controls all of our automatic behaviors and body processes, including metabolism, digestion, and weight loss or gain, she would probably continue to fail until her subconscious agreed with the idea.

We decided to use hypnosis to find out the reason why her subconscious refused to lose weight. Once in trance, we went back in time to the moment this decision to be overweight was made. Karen saw herself as a little five-year-old girl. She was with her mom, standing by her grandmother's bed. Karen remembered feeling very sad and scared as she looked at her emaciated granny. She looked almost like a skeleton as she slept under the effects of the pain killers. Her mother said as she sobbed, "Poor Mom, she lost more weight, she is so thin, she will die soon." Karen's grandmother died of cancer, but in her five-year-old mind, she died of losing weight, of becoming thin.

We processed Karen's five-year-old's fears and the decision she made at that time to hold on to weight in order to stay alive by looking at them through her adult understanding. Now it all made sense. Our subconscious mind always wants the best for us, but we need to remember that it does not always know what the best is. The subconscious makes decisions and forms ideas at a young age, from phrases said by authority figures, from deep experiences we do not fully understand at that age. It formulates commandments that will guide our life even if it drives us to failure or suffering in an attempt to protect us from "a worse evil," in Karen's case, dying of losing weight. The beauty of this is that once we understand, once we see the origin of that mistaken commandment and correct it, everything becomes amazingly easy because, as we said, our subconscious wants the best for us, it just needs to know what the best is.

Karen is now enjoying a life free of freedom from a protection she didn't need and one that was ruining her life. She is happily and safely losing weight.

Hypnosis is just one of the tools that can be used when removing imprints. An imprint is something we heard from an authority figure under an emotionally charged state, which is stored in our minds as a law or mandate. In Karen's case, "losing weight will kill you." It usually happens when we are very young, and we never question or review it. Moreover, we are not even aware of its existence. Unless we bring it to awareness and deactivate it, we will be like a puppet whose movements are run by the threads of the imprints. There are many other tools that can also be effective in finding and removing imprints. Therapy, journaling, meditation, and awareness are all useful and effective. You need to find the one that works for you. You can do it with professional help, and you can also do it by seriously engaging in the task of observing and questioning yourself. "What would I be feeling now if I weren't feeling hungry?" is a good question to ask. Once you get an answer, you can deal with that feeling much more effectively than by covering it with food. Be gentle but relentless with yourself. Keep in mind that even your most destructive behaviors are an attempt to provide a response to a need, like in Karen's case. But at the same time be relentless in evaluating what the real need is and what the appropriate response for your ultimate good is.

Another useful tool in the taming of your subconscious is to *increase self-esteem*. When you listen to someone talk, if you listen attentively, you will find out that the solution to his or her problem is right there, in the wording of the problem itself. How many times have you heard or even said, "He/she has let me down?" Now open your ears, your mind's ears, and listen again. What are you really saying? You are saying that you have placed yourself in a position where someone else had to hold you up. You have given away your power. You have renounced your ability to choose. If you had retained your power instead, if you had exercised your ability to make choices, no one else would be holding you. You wouldn't need that. Instead, you would be up on your own, self-sustained, solidly standing on your own strength. And what happens when you are in such a position of self-strength? First, you are in control of your destiny. Second, you can relate to others from a place of freedom, not one of need. You can choose to be with someone because you want, not out of fear that they might drop you and you would be let down.

Metaphors are the language of the unconscious. They are a wonderful gateway to understanding our deeper selves. When we translate our inner world into language, the words we use are not random. There is a deeper layer of meaning that we often miss. By repeating the phrase over and over, by hearing it so often, our conscious minds have come to forget its primitive meaning. But our unconscious still remembers, so choose the words you speak wisely.

Give it a try; start exercising the muscles of your mind's ear. Listen to your choice of words, and use that clue to arrive at a better understanding of yourself. The solution to your problem is right there, just waiting to be heard.

So, if you are one of these people that often feel you were let down, try this exercise in a quiet place and time for yourself (please, never ever while driving):

1. Sit on a comfortable chair (phones turned off), with your back straight, legs uncrossed, feet on the floor. Close your eyes.
2. Take a few deep breaths.
3. Imagine you are a strong tree. Visualize your roots going down from the plant of your feet, deep into the earth, and your branches and leaves, green and healthy, reaching up to the sky. Feel yourself grounded, rooted, so solidly planted that you can now reach up and grow confidently to the height you want.

Another thing to keep in mind is that if you want to be fit, you must learn to speak, to *use the proper language*. Every time you talk or think about "losing weight" your subconscious shrieks. Nobody likes "to lose," nobody wants to "be a loser." These terms have negative unconscious associations. Try thinking and talking about "being fit" or "achieving your perfect weight." Now you have many more chances of enlisting help from your subconscious. The other important concept is that your subconscious does not "read" the word "no." When you tell yourself, "I will not eat bread at my lunch meeting," your subconscious reads, "Eat bread," and that's all you can think of. Bread seems to pop up from the background like a neon sign. If I now ask you not to think about a pink elephant, all that will come to your mind is a pink elephant, even though before I said it a pink elephant was not even remotely in your mind. So, if you tell yourself, "I will eat a nice salad" or "I will make vegetables the most important part of my meal," your internal radar will be focusing on detecting salads and vegetables and bringing that to your attention.

Increasing your self esteem and using the proper language are very helpful, and *defining your goal* is paramount. How will you know how to get there if you don't know what "there" is like? Have you ever wondered why some people get what they want so easily, as if good things just happen to fall on their lap, while others constantly struggle as if they'd be swimming against the tide?

Your unconscious mind has a radar, and it is ready to work with you if you would only know how to input the right coordinates. We often say, "I want to be happy" or "I want to be successful." And, although these are genuine desires, they are so vague that they become meaningless. Moreover, they don't provide your unconscious mind with any destination. How are you supposed to make a route map if you don't know where you are going?

Discouraged? Relax, this is easy to solve and you can start working on it now by applying these tips. Start by imagining what your life would be like if you had already achieved your goal. What will life be like once you are at your ideal weight? Be specific; visualize what you would be doing, how a whole day in your life would be from the moment you wake up. Use as many details as possible. What clothes are you wearing? What are your surroundings like? What sounds can you hear? Do you recognize any smell? How would those around you know that you have achieved that desired state? What would they notice about you that's different? What would change at work? Home? Socially?

Be consistent in practicing this on a daily basis. Your unconscious mind understands by repetition. The more you rehearse this in the theater of your mind, the more consistent reactions you will spontaneously experience. By doing this over and over, your inner route map will naturally adapt. Remember that the more vividly you experience these images in your mind, the easier it is for your unconscious mind to drive your actions in a manner consistent with that goal. Thoughts are energy, and that energy can take different forms and materialize. Have you ever experienced salivating when thinking about your favorite food? Well, your imagination has elicited that response. You can elicit different actions and reactions by thinking the right kind of thoughts.

Now, a word of caution: Unless you believe that you deserve that goal and have the ability to achieve it, you won't move in that direction. Your self-image is like your point of reference that tells your unconscious which destinations are open. If you believe you are a shmuck, you will get shmucky results. Maybe it's time to start reviewing what you truly and deeply believe about yourself. Do you "deserve" to be thin and feel gorgeous? Imagine yourself being already at the desired weight and looking attractive. How do you feel? If you have any feeling of discomfort, it's time to check your belief system about your looks. Are you afraid of attracting other men and being tempted to have an affair? Have you been told that your role in the family is to be kind and sweet, but not pretty? Would anyone around you feel threatened by your being more attractive? Are you "not supposed" to overshadow someone else in your family? Do you feel guilty about becoming more attractive than your mother/daughter/sister? Where did you get the idea that this is a competition? How would shining in all your splendor affect others you love? These are all questions you need to reflect upon if you get any sort of discomfort while imagining yourself fit and thin. If you don't get a good warm happy feeling when you picture yourself that way, it means the saboteur has been invited to the party. I invite you to meditate on the following writing by Marianne Williamson, who has so beautifully addressed this fear:

> "Our deepest fear is not that we are inadequate. Our deepest fear is that we are powerful beyond measure. It is our light, not our darkness that most frightens us. We ask ourselves, "Who am I to be brilliant, gorgeous, talented, fabulous?" Actually, who are you not to be? You are a child of God. Your playing small does not serve the world. There is nothing enlightened about shrinking so that other people won't feel insecure around you. We are all meant to shine, as children do. We were born to make manifest the glory of God that is within us. It's not just in some of us; it's in everyone. And as we let our own light shine, we unconsciously give other people permission to do the same. As we are liberated from our own fear, our presence automatically liberates others.

Secret #10:

A deeper look at the golden rule

A man came into my office looking gloomy, exhausted, and stressed. I asked the usual questions about his lifestyle and diet. He said he slept four to five hours. His breakfast was bottled orange juice, frozen pancakes with syrup, sometimes eggs if he had time, and two cups of coffee. For lunch, he usually had a sandwich or a Caesar salad with "a lot" of dressing, and a croissant or doughnut with coffee in the afternoon. He loved pasta for dinner or a juicy steak with potatoes, and then some Oreo cookies and milk while watching TV. He did not like vegetables other than potatoes, and as to fruits, only if they had cream and sugar or were canned with syrup. Exercise? No…there was no time for that. Stress management? Relaxation? No…that was for wimps. Last checkup? He couldn't remember.

"Now let me ask some questions about your car," I said. He looked at me as if I had just landed from Mars. "Let's suppose you decide to go on a road trip. Four hours after you start, you see a red light in your panel saying "check engine," would you continue driving for the rest of the trip? "Of course not," he said, "I'd get off the road and look for a mechanic as soon as possible." "Now imagine that in this town there is a very fancy gas station right across from the mechanic," I continued. "They sell a new gasoline that comes in different colors and smells—designer perfume gas—and you can choose from Armani, Burberry, Fendi, Hugo Boss, and so on. They advertise on TV, magazines…everywhere, so you've seen the commercials many times. You ask the mechanic about it and he tells you that it's really poor quality fuel. Your car will drive, but after a while, it will damage the engine. Would you put that fuel in your car?" I asked him. "Of course not," he said with a note of indignation in his voice like the mere thought of doing that to his car was unacceptable…and after a few seconds he realized.

"Yes," I said. "You will not force your car to drive when something is going wrong and you will stop to fix it, even if that causes a small delay in your road trip. You will only give it quality fuel regardless of the smell, appearance, or advertising. Then why do you put any sort of adulterated low quality fuel in your body, just because it's easy and tastes good? Why do you force your body to keep going when it is telling you something needs attention? If your car breaks down you can always get a replacement. Unfortunately, your body is the only vehicle you get for the journey in this lifetime. If you want a long and pleasurable ride…you'd better start taking care of it. Do onto you as you do onto your car."

"Love your neighbor like yourself"…we've heard it hundreds of times. We usually focus on the "love your neighbor" part, but we miss the notion upon which this rule has been conceived: You must first love yourself. How can you give someone else something you don't have in you? This rule that has transcended place and time can only be implemented provided we first learn to love ourselves. When you love yourself, it becomes easy and natural to want the best for you. Taking care of yourself no longer produces guilt or discomfort. Excuses that justify ignoring your needs vanish. You make friends with the idea that you deserve the best, until it goes from an idea to certainty.

If you had a very important guest in your home, wouldn't you want your house to look its best? You'd probably clean it, get rid of the clutter on the table, light candles, and maybe buy flowers. You wouldn't think of serving a bag of chips or TV microwave dinner; you would cook a special meal, do anything you can to make him or her comfortable and honored, wouldn't you? Well, you do have a special guest—you have a soul, a spark of God, a slice of the collective consciousness, or any other name you want to call it... inside of you. What holds you together? What makes you remain "you" in spite of the fact that each and every cell in your body dies and is replaced by a new one all the time? Who could be a more important guest than that? Wouldn't you want to make this guest feel comfortable and honored? Be a good host; make your body and your mind a clean, uncluttered, comfortable, and cozy home for your most important guest!

Meditation is a great way to connect with our *wise self*, to recover that feeling of love and acceptance. Meditation does not have to be a difficult process or something destined to special people. You don't need to be a yogi or a Tibetan monk. Moreover, you probably meditate somehow in your own way, every time you daydream or focus intensively in a thought, image, or idea. Some people call it active visualization, others self-hypnosis. Regardless of what you call it, the process of taking some time in silence and solitude to go inside and reflect, to focus on images and feelings, can make a ground-breaking difference in your life. Here are some ideas on loving meditation:

1. Sit in a quiet place, in silence. Focus your mind on someone you love—your children, your spouse, your grandmother. It doesn't even matter if the person is still alive. It can even be someone you don't personally know, but you deeply respect and admire, someone you love. As you focus your mind on that person, notice the warmth on your body. Imagine that the feeling of love is now a light that is shinning on that person. What color is that light? Now make the beam of light larger and larger until you are also immersed in that light. Let that light shine all around you and inside of you, filling every cell, every tissue, and every organ of your body. Stay there, absorbing that love, bathing in it, and becoming that love. Slowly, when you are ready, return your attention to the room, to the now, bringing the love with you; and, when you are ready, open your eyes.

2. Go out to a garden or park and look around. Notice the beauty of nature. Chose a flower and take a closer look. Admire the color, the texture, the intricate patterns of its design. Now think about the intelligence that flows underneath, that makes it transform sunlight into energy, that absorbs nutrients from the soil. Picture the cells that form that flower working together in harmony. Sense the life force in it. Take a moment to admire that expression of life, notice how it is perfect just as it is. Would you challenge or question anything about it? Now take a moment to identify that same life force, that same harmony, that same perfection in yourself. Notice if there is any resistance to looking and accepting your right to exist, your own beauty and perfection. Allow the resistance to vanish as you focus

only on the life force running through you, just as it runs through that flower.

3.   Deepak Chopra, in *The Book of Secrets*, shares this meditation for unity and love: Lay on the floor, close your eyes and take a deep breath. Notice how the air feels going deeply inside and follow the sensation as it slowly comes out. Think of the room around you and say to yourself, "I am not in this room, this room is in me." Now expand your awareness to the house or building and say, "I am not in this house/building. This building is in me." Now expand your awareness to your neighborhood and say, "I am not in this neighborhood, this neighborhood is in me." Now picture your city and say, "I am not in this city. This city is in me." Now think of your country and say, "I am not in this country. This country is in me." Now make a mental picture of the continent and say, "I am not in this continent. This continent is in me." Now visualize the world, with its oceans, countries, mountains, and people, and say, "I am not in this world. This world is in me." Now expand even further and visualize or think of the universe and say, "I am not in this universe. This universe is in me." Take a few moments to focus on that notion, on that feeling, and slowly return your awareness to the room. At your own time, open your eyes.

4.   Sit in a quiet place in silence. Ground yourself by breathing slowly, deeply, and rhythmically, following the path of the air into your nose lungs, the oxygen reaching your organs and tissues, allowing them to become more comfortable and relaxed. Imagine yourself sitting in a room. Notice what the room looks like. The room has a large glass window. Now think of someone in your life that loves you deeply and unconditionally, whether that person is still alive or not. Picture that person looking at you through that glass window. Let a part of you float out of your body

that is sitting in the room and drift toward the person looking at you. Look into his/her eyes and pay attention to the
expression of love in them. Now float into that person and
look at yourself sitting in that room. Look from within that
person. Feel what it is like to look at yourself with total un-
limited unconditional love. Absorb that love, allow yourself
to soak in that love, capture it. Now float out of that person
and drift back into your body bringing with you a part of
that love. Take a deep breath, and slowly open your eyes.

In all these meditations, it is a good practice to write down
any feelings or ideas that arise immediately after doing them. You
can rotate them, and notice if the feelings change as you continue
practicing them.

In addition to meditations, you may also want to experiment
with affirmations. The important point when working with affirmations is noticing how you feel as you say them to yourself. The way
you feel, the emotions that arise, the inner voice that contests or
answers the affirmation gives you important information and ele-
ments to work on. If you tell yourself, "I can do this," and a voice
inside says, "Yeah…like the last time you tried?" it is time to work
on your beliefs. Again, be gentle and relentless. Don't judge yourself; just observe, follow the voice, and see where it comes from.
Find reasons to dispute it, to prove it wrong. Find examples of other
times or situations when you succeeded at something, even if it is
completely unrelated. If you succeeded at something, even if it is
learning to ride a bicycle or graduating from elementary school,
you have the germ of success inside of you. And you can transfer it
to other areas. Think about something difficult you mastered, like
moving, raising your kids, surviving a divorce, finishing that proj-
ect. What resources did you use then? You still have those resources
in you. It's like learning a language; once you learn it, you learn it.

If you can speak French in the living room, you can also speak it in the kitchen. Dispute that damn negative deprecating voice with all your might and prove it wrong. Assert your right to live well. That right belongs to you for the mere reason that you exist, and no matter what, it's yours.

Here is an affirmation you can repeat silently before putting anything in your mouth. This will remind you of your goal and strengthen your commitment. Make it your silent prayer or sing it, or say it in your own words:

"From now on, I only feed my body what my body needs, rather than what my mind thinks it wants. I choose the permanent satisfaction of my perfect body over the momentary pleasure of my taste buds. This is my pledge to myself: To honor, love, and respect my being, to take care of my real rather than my imaginary needs, to listen to my wise self, remembering it is a divine spark that resides in me."

Besides the "before eating or drinking" affirmation, below is a list of daily reflections to help you through the first three months of your new way of relating to food. As we discussed before, it takes an average of three months until a new behavior becomes a habit. So use all the support you can give yourself during this period. These affirmations and reflections will help you to stay focused and remain on track. Choose one phrase daily and carry it with you throughout your day. Copy them into your journal, email them to yourself, or write them down on a Post-it note or index card. Meditate on them and discuss them with friends, family, or coworkers. They are a great tool to help you reach your weight goals!

1. If you want pleasure hug someone...food is for nourishment.
2. "Let food be your medicine and medicine your food" (Hippocrates).

3. Which pleasure lasts longer, the taste of a piece of candy or the satisfaction of looking gorgeous?

4. More disease is created through excess eating than through lack.

5. Your body is a temple, not a trashcan or a storage container. When you've had enough, throw the rest in the proper trashcan or store it in the refrigerator.

6. Remember, there is plenty of food available at all times; you don't need to carry an extra supply in your body.

7. Before you eat, always ask yourself, "What do I really need now?"

8. We are mostly water; we need water more than we need food. Drink a glass of water when you feel hungry and more often than not, you will feel satisfied.

9. Repeat to yourself, "I will stick to my goal. I will be victorious."

10. Cravings are nothing more than habits. A bad habit can be easily replaced with a good one.

11. You have already been successful in something. Make a list of your past successes, write next to each what qualities or resources you applied and then think how you can apply the same to achieve your fitness goal.

12. Anything that another person has achieved is achievable. If other people have been able to attain their perfect weight, so can you.

13. Love yourself, and the world will love you. Treat yourself with respect and the world will respect you. When you are about to eat ask yourself, "Am I showing love and respect to myself through this food choice?"

14. When you are hungry between meals, think that it's your body getting rid of excess fat, it's a way of getting closer to your goal; you are safe and you are OK.

15. Thank your body and appreciate the message it is communicating instead of ruining it with unnecessary food.
16. You are what you eat. Eat well.
17. You wouldn't think of eating poison, would you? Refined sugar is poison.
18. Breathe deeply and slowly, counting to four when you inhale and eight when you exhale. Do that ten times before you eat so you are centered and calm and you can listen to what your body needs.
19. Eat only when you are calm, never when you are angry or upset. You don't want to ingest and store anger; you want to get rid of it.
20. If you are anxious, breathe, walk, talk to a friend, or write down your thoughts about being anxious. Don't eat; it will only increase your anxiety by adding guilt.
21. Every time you have made a good choice regarding food, you are closer to success; you are building a memory of success. Appreciate yourself for that. Be proud of yourself. Say it to yourself.
22. Make a list of rewards that are not food related, like a foot massage, a new CD or book, a pleasant scent, time for yourself. Think of at least ten ideas to reward yourself and do it every day you have stuck to your goal.
23. Make a list of things that soothe you or help you process negative feelings that are not food related. Write them down; keep them handy.
24. You can change a negative thought by thinking a positive one. Your brain cannot think two opposite thoughts at the same time, so, it's your choice.
25. When you think, "I've had a rough day; I deserve some ice cream/cookie/comfort food," ask yourself how that is

going to help you feel better. How will you really feel after you've had it? How will that solve your problem?

26. Would you do something to harm your child? Why would you act different toward your inner child? Your inner child wants love, not carbohydrates.

27. Close your eyes and picture yourself bathed in a golden healing light. See your stress melting away…feel the warmth…take a few deep breaths. Do this every time you need to calm down.

28. Imagine you are wearing a magic contact lens that lets you see food for what it really is. When you look at white bread, candy, cookies, cakes, or any refined sugar, you will see the real thing—a pile of yellowish fat that will sabotage your goal if you eat it.

29. You can choose to remember what you know. You have enough nutritional information to avoid bread, sugars, and excess fat. Before you put a bite in your mouth say, "I choose to remember."

30. Artificial sweeteners won't help you lose weight; they jeopardize your health by sending wrong signals to your brain. Choose moderate amounts of natural products.

31. Water is your best friend; we are mostly made of water. We come from water, not sodas! Drink water; forget sodas, even if they are "diet" or "light." Every time you drink soda or coffee, you are missing an opportunity to drink water. Water cleanses your system. A clean system can better regulate metabolism and get rid of toxins and fat deposits.

32. Life is movement…why drive around in circles trying to save steps? Park far, take the opportunity to walk, use the stairs, move, and be alive. A butt that moves stays young.

33. Digestion starts in your mouth; chew your food thoroughly. Your stomach will thank you by staying flat instead of bloated.

34. Your taste buds are in your mouth, the more you chew food, the more pleasure you get from it. If you swallow without chewing, you are introducing calories without even getting any satisfaction. Why would you want to eat fast?

35. It takes approximately twenty minutes for your brain to get the signal that you've had enough food. If you gulp food like a caveman, by the time your brain gets the stop sign you've already stuffed yourself. SLOW DOWN!

36. Eat only sitting at the table, with proper setting and plates. Your meal is a sensory experience; savor it in a relaxed environment. If you are stressed or in a rush, wait until you can eat like this.

37. Don't eat in your car, or standing in front of the refrigerator, or while working on the computer, or watching TV. If you do that, you won't even notice you are eating, much less *how much* you are eating, and you'll be hungry shortly afterwards.

38. Once you've made the habit of eating only when sitting properly at the table, you will notice you don't snack as much. Your mind will stop calling for food when doing other things. You are a creature of habit. Get good habits.

39. Take a moment to thank the universe for the food you are about to eat. It will transform the action into a spiritual experience.

40. Choose natural products, the less processed a food, the better for your body. Nature is wise. Follow it; listen to it.

41. The whiter the bread the sooner you're dead. Whole grains have micronutrients and vitamins. Why would you want to throw them away and eat the garbage left?

42. An apple a day keeps the doctor away…or any other fruit. Next time you want candy or cookies, eat a piece of fruit instead, and think of all the wonderful nutrients you are getting; feel yourself becoming healthier.

43. Find ways to reward yourself that have nothing to do with food. Make a list. Pamper yourself the good way.

44. Learn to do the "thank yourself meditation." Thank yourself for everything you do that's good for you. You brushed your teeth? Say, "Thank you (your name) for keeping your teeth clean and healthy." You cleaned your house? Thank yourself. You listened to a friend? Thank yourself. Use every opportunity to acknowledge and honor yourself, and you will notice your confidence growing.

45. Learn to breathe deeply. Imagine a balloon in your belly inflating every time you breathe in, and deflating every time you breathe out. Do it slowly, like a baby sleeping, and you'll feel peaceful as one.

46. Orchids, one of the most beautiful flowers, live only and exclusively on water and air. Learn from the orchid; your main focus is enough water and proper breathing.

47. Learn to develop self-acceptance. You need to accept where you are in order to start your process of improvement. Stand in front of a mirror, naked (yes, I don't care how hard it is) and thank every part of your body for what it does for you. Say it out loud, "Thank you feet for walking me around…thank you legs for carrying me…thank you butt for cushioning my bones when I sit, and so on. It is easier to take care of something you value than something you despise. Every part of your body is valuable.

48. Learn and incorporate these magic words, "I now choose to…" Feeling calm and centered is a choice. Eating healthy is a choice. Overcoming a craving is a choice. Being motivated is a choice. Choose!

49. Stay away from bad influences; you don't want to go out to eat with a saboteur. Go out to eat with people who are role models for how you want to look and behave. Make

fit friends, observe them in action, copy them, and model yourself after them.

50. Learn to say no without guilt. The next time your mom or neighbor says, "Just eat one; it won't do you any harm" or "I made them for you," say, "Thank you, I'll take one for later," and throw it away before you change your mind. Or say "I won't have it for health reasons" or "Thank you so much. I value your gesture, even if I don't eat it." Practice this; find an answer that feels right. Your goal is more important than being a people's pleaser.

51. You are a wonderful creation of the universe. You deserve to be healthy. You deserve to look and feel great. Putting yourself down doesn't help you or the world. Taking care of yourself is your best contribution to humanity.

52. Supermodels are made of the same material as you are. You can choose to look and feel like one.

53. When you see, think, or smell food, it is a stimulus. Your behavior is the reaction to that stimulus. Your goal is to expand the space between the stimuli and the reaction. It is in that space where you decide what's best for you. It is in that space where freedom resides. Any reaction without stopping in that space is slavery, is being a robot. Be free, learning to expand the moment between the stimuli and your reaction. The more time you spend in that space, the better choice you'll make.

54. Proper weight is a result of good health. Think healthy, act healthy, and you'll be healthy...and gorgeous.

55. Nature is on your side. Your body tends to balance naturally. You just need to remove the obstacles and it will get rid of any excess.

56. In order to function properly, your metabolism needs proper rest. Adequate sleep is essential to achieve your ideal weight.

57. You need both movement and rest in the right balance. Too much of a good thing can become bad.

58. Learn from children; let exercise be fun. Play! Once you get used to exercising, you will actually enjoy it.

59. Laughing is a great aid for good health and proper weight. When you laugh, your brain secretes hormones that make you feel good. When you feel good, it's easier to choose what's best. Laugh! It feels great and it's free.

60. Don't do to yourself what you wouldn't do to your loved ones. Would you cover your ears or turn around when someone you love is talking? Be kind to yourself. Listen to your body and treat it with respect.

61. Portion control is one of your best tools. When you go to a restaurant, order a "take out" container at the same time you order your food. Take half of your food, place it in the container, close it, and put it in the bag. Or share with someone else. Your food shouldn't be larger than your hand. That's all you need.

62. Be creative; make your plate a colorful vegetable master-piece. Spend a moment admiring it as you would do with a painting or a sculpture. Involve all your senses in the expe-rience, not just the taste.

63. Today, play a game with your kids or a friend: take turns naming a vegetable or fruit. The last one to come up with a name wins. You will be surprised at how much variety exists…and you may be tempted to try one.

64. Take a moment to thank your body for what it does for you, regardless of its shape or volume. Think of all the places your legs take you to, all the people your arms allow you to hug.

65. You have a right to be happy.

66. Be like the ameba; walk away from what is bad for you, and move closer to what is good.

67. If you cover your emotions with food, they will still be there, and find a way out. It has happened before, and you know it.

68. Find a non-food related social activity and invite a friend to join you.

69. Have you stopped today to take a look at the color of the sky?

70. Spend a moment visualizing yourself in your perfect weight; notice how you feel.

71. What would you be thinking about if you were not thinking about food or weight?

72. You cannot control the way others feel. When someone you care about is in pain or distress, you are not personally responsible.

73. Do you feel threatened when others get close?

74. Food is not an anesthetic. Food is food.

75. Are you eating because you are anxious about having eaten?

76. A nutritional plan is not a punishment. It is a choice.

77. Write three additional ways of rewarding yourself that are not food related.

78. Cravings are messengers. Listen closely to the message. What is behind the craving? What do you really need?

79. You are always in the right place and at the right moment, even if it is challenging or painful. You don't have to like the situation but you have to accept it as part of your reality.

80. Where did you get the idea that you have to feel good all the time?

90. Sit with your feelings. Don't be afraid of them. They will not destroy you; they just want you to listen, that's all.

91. Be assertive. Say what you need to say. What is it that you need to communicate right now?

92. Remind yourself of why you want to be fit.

93. What does spirituality mean to you? How are you experiencing your spirituality?

94. Being "over-busy" is a close relative of "over-eating."

95. Take responsibility for yourself and your feelings, and not for everyone else and their feelings. This is not being selfish; it's being realistic.

96. When your actions are aligned with who you are and what you believe in, things flow.

97. Are you eating out of control because you cannot control the way others around you act or feel?

98. If anyone hurt you, shame on them. Don't punish yourself with excess food.

99. Are you being honest with yourself?

100. Make a list of activities you can do instead of bingeing. When the urge to binge strikes, tell yourself you will make a decision whether to eat or not, only *after* you have done one of the activities in your list.

Epilogue

A s the Green Fairy handed over the manuscript to the trembling hands of the President of the Wisdom Council, she said, "Unfortunately (or not), this time you cannot take care of doing this for the princess. She needs to do it by herself. All you can do is deliver the manuscript and wait." The Green Fairy made a circular movement over her head with her right hand, and began to turn more and more ethereal, vanishing from the feet up, soon leaving nothing behind but a transparent sparkly green dust in the air, and a hint of her garden scent.

When Princess Sandra retired to her bedroom that evening, she found a package on her bed, wrapped with a green ribbon and a card. She looked at it with a hopeless sigh of indifference, assuming it was another attempt from her parents to cheer her up with more stuff. But something in that ribbon was different, special. She picked up the package and opened the note, which read, "This is the missing gift...sorry for the delay. Yours, Green Fairy." The princess felt a bite of curiosity that she had not felt in years as she tore the wrapping paper. She sat on her bed, with the manuscript in her hands, and started reading; she read all night long, only stopping to wipe the tears rolling down her eyes.

In the days that followed, Princess Sandra was seen at all times carrying a notebook and a pen. She would often stop on her steps and stay very still, sometimes with her eyes closed, for a few moments, before smiling as she wrote something in her notebook.

The king and queen witnessed in astonished joy all the changes that took place for months. Sandra discovered a passion for dancing. She stopped using her self-upgrading phone to call the kitchen and instead started to walk there and personally choose. She found out that she has fun cooking and channels her artistic talent into preparing colorful salads and creative fresh dishes. She made an organic vegetable garden that is her pride and hobby, where she enjoys dipping her hands in the earth, breathing in the green smell, and sweating as she takes care of tomatoes, lettuces, spinach, radishes and so many other beautiful vegetables. She donated the winged horse chariot to charity and now rides a bicycle to the mall (OK, yes, her aids still pick up her shopping bags and take them to the palace for her). She shed the excess pounds and achieved her perfect weight. Perfect, because it's the one that makes her happy, full of energy, content in her own skin, and healthy in mind and body. Sandra didn't merely shed pounds; she got rid of the heavy baggage she was carrying for years—all those buried emotions, all those unmet needs that were so difficult to admit and look at. As her fat melted, so did her isolation, her challenges to make real contact with others and cultivate relationships. Sandra became mindful of her thoughts and feelings and learned to take time to check with herself.

Princess Sandra now enjoys a different kind of food and appreciates what it does for her health rather than her taste buds. The king and queen are no longer worried about finding a husband for her; they know that as Princess Sandra learns to love herself, she will soon find someone special to love as well. As Sandra becomes more and more aware of her needs, she also will develop the ability to communicate effectively and stand her ground, kindly and firmly. The Wisdom Council recently voted and signed an amendment to the rules that stipulated a marring age for princesses. They all agree that when the moment comes, Sandra will be very qualified to rule, with or without a prince. Anyhow, considering the glow in her face and the liveliness of her eyes, I would not be surprised to hear bells soon.

The End

Appendix A: Thin Ever After eating plan

The Thin Ever After eating plan is a flexible, easy to do, "pick and chose" tool. The purpose is to give you ideas, which you can customize into your personal plan. As we discussed in Secret #7, planning ahead of time is one of the keys to success. Some diet plans give you a structured day-by-day, meal-by-meal plan. If you are (like me), opinionated and like to be in control (Who said anything about control freak?), you may feel trapped with that kind of plan, and resent the fact that you have no say in the matter. Also, if you eat out a lot, it may be challenging. That's why this plan only gives you options and ideas. You chose what and when. Below you will find a list of sensible, success supportive breakfasts, lunches, dinners, and snacks. Feel free to make your own mix, or use them to get inspired when you don't know what to eat.

Notes:

- In all meat dishes, try to use grass fed, hormone and antibiotic free meat.
- In all chicken dishes, try to use hormone and antibiotic free chicken.
- Chose hormone and antibiotic free eggs. When eating eggs for breakfast, don't chose a lunch or snack with eggs. Eggs are good, but don't overdo—maximum of two per day, preferable one whole and one egg white.
- If you can only buy some organic produce, chose apples, spinach, berries, and celery, which are more heavily sprayed or difficult to brush.
- When using cold cuts, chose nitrate and preservative free.

- Drink plenty of fresh water between meals, avoid sodas, limit alcohol to one glass of wine no more than three times a week.

- Limit coffee to one cup per day; feel free to drink as much herbal teas as desired. Remember, coffee is very acidic and affects the alkaline acid balance in your body.

- You can make cranberry water (great to get rid of water retained in tissues) by diluting one glass of unsweetened cranberry juice in four glasses of water. Add the juice of a fresh lemon and season with stevia, cinnamon, and a dash of cayenne for an extra metabolism boost and toxin burning.

- Dress salads with one tablespoon of olive oil and balsamic or apple cider vinegar or lemon. Don't overdo with salt, it causes water retention. When possible, use unprocessed sea salt.

- Use frozen vegetables or fruits freely, just make sure the only ingredients are the vegetables or fruits, and nothing added (no sauce, dressings, or sugar).

- Eat mindfully; enjoying the scent, colors, texture and taste. Pay attention to your eating and avoid TV, reading, or stressful conversations. If you are distracted, you won't register the food you ingested and will feel hungry sooner. Once you finish eating, if you are home, brush your teeth to signal the end of that meal.

Breakfast options

1. Protein fiber pancake: Mix 1 scoop of whey protein powder, 1 egg and 1 egg white, cinnamon, and ½ cup of Fiber One original cereal in a bowl. Cook in a pan in medium heat for only a couple of minutes each side. You can put blueberries and a little agave on top after it's done.

2. Mango-Berry smoothie: Put ½ cup of frozen mango and ½ cup of frozen berries in the blender, add ½ cup of plain

organic yogurt, 1 tablespoon of chia seeds, a little stevia, and cinnamon; blend till smoothilicious!

3. Combine 1 cup of plain cooked oatmeal with ¼ cup of sunflower seeds. Use stevia or agave to sweeten.

4. Peel and chop 1 apple; add a little honey, the juice of half a lemon, ¼ cup of raisins and cinnamon. Cook in microwave for one minute, and delight in the smell and taste…nothing to envy from an apple pie!

5. On 2 slices of Ezekiel bread, spread 1 tablespoon (one for both slices) of almond butter or organic peanut butter.

6. Scrambled 2 eggs with vegetables (onions, peppers, spinach, mushrooms, and anything green you can think of).

7. For an asparagus and scallion omelet with goat cheese, use two eggs and ¼ cup goat cheese.

8. Try 2 eggs over easy with a scoop of salsa on top, and 1 slice of Ezekiel bread.

9. Mix 1 cup plain organic Greek yogurt with ½ cup of blueberries, ¼ cup of chopped raw walnuts, cinnamon, and stevia to taste.

10. A nice bowl of fresh fruit with ¼ cup of chopped raw almonds and pumpkin seeds makes a nice breakfast.

11. Try 5 slices of nitrate-free turkey rolled over slices from half an avocado.

12. For tofu egg salad, mix ¼ of the tofu package with minced scallions, celery, lemon juice, 2 tablespoons of organic mayonnaise, Dijon mustard, turmeric, and a dash of cayenne pepper.

13. To make a berry protein shake, blend 1 cup of frozen berries, 1 scoop of whey protein, and fresh water (add until desired consistency).

14. For a "Nutty Banana," roll a peeled banana on thinly chopped raw nuts and then cut in slices.

15. A breakfast sandwich made by filling a toasted whole grain English muffin with a slice of avocado, tomato, sprouts,

goat cheese and a dash of balsamic vinegar is a nice start to the day.

16. Homemade hummus on whole grain pita is very healthy. To make hummus, smash or process chickpeas with a little olive oil, garlic, sea salt and pepper.
17. Why not just a delicious crunchy apple today?
18. Chicken leftovers wrapped on lettuce leaves are an easy fix.
19. Try ½ cup cooked natural oatmeal with 1 chopped apple, a few walnuts, cinnamon, and agave to taste.
20. Try 1 cup pineapple chunks and ¼ cup raw sunflower seeds.
21. You might enjoy 2 poached eggs with salsa.

Lunch options

1. For salmon salad, combine 1 can wild salmon, mixed greens, tomatoes, onions, cucumbers, peppers, and dress with the juice of half a fresh lemon, a little dijon mustard, 1 tablespoon olive oil, and apple cider vinegar.
2. Try a turkey and avocado sandwich with sprouted bread.
3. Greek salad (lettuce, tomatoes, black olives, onions, and feta cheese) dressed with 1 tablespoon olive oil, balsamic vinegar, and ground kelp is a tasty option.
4. Spinach, goat cheese, and walnut salad is another tasty salad.
5. Mix and spread 2 boiled eggs, half a chopped onion, 1 tablespoon organic mayonnaise, and capers over half a whole grain bagel (only if you didn't have eggs for breakfast).
6. Chopped chicken leftovers over arugula and spinach and dressed with one tablespoon olive oil and apple cider vinegar makes a tasty salad option.
7. Quinoa salad is made with 1 cup cooked quinoa with chopped scallions, peppers, tomatoes, cucumbers and cabbage.

8. Try 1 can of sardines over shredded purple and green cabbage, shredded carrots with fresh lemon juice, and 1 tablespoon organic mayonnaise.

9. Sprouted lentil salad (Whole Foods now sells dried sprouted lentils and you only need to soak them for twenty minutes to rehydrate, no cooking necessary) with chopped veggies is delicious.

10. Try sprouted mung beans (same instructions as 9, above) and mashed squash (you can buy it frozen and thaw in microwave).

11. A hummus, spinach, and sprouts wrap is an easy fix.

12. Frozen mixed vegetables (like broccoli, carrots and cauliflower), cooked on the stovetop on medium low with a little water, turmeric, basil, kelp and sea salt, and any protein leftover full of good nutrients.

13. Try a nitrate-free turkey, lettuce, and tomato sandwich with mustard.

14. Combine mashed sardines with fresh lemon juice and a little organic mayonnaise and sprouts, then wrap in lettuce leaves or a whole grain wrap.

15. For a cobb salad, combine chopped chicken, a hardboiled egg, mixed greens, bleu cheese, and tomatoes, and dress with olive oil and vinegar.

16. For salmon nicoise, combine 1 can of wild salmon, boiled and cubed potatoes, mixed greens, sun-dried tomatoes, and green beans.

17. Make a chef's salad with roast beef, one slice of Swiss cheese, a hardboiled egg, mixed greens, and tomato with olive oil and vinegar.

18. Try a homemade hamburger with tomato and lettuce on a whole grain thin bun

19. Try a grilled portobello mushroom, eggplant, and pepper sandwich

20. Grilled seasoned tofu (basil, oregano, pepper, turmeric) on mixed greens, spinach, shredded carrot, and tomato with olive oil and vinegar makes a great salad.

21. Beefsteak tomato stuffed with salmon salad (made with wild canned salmon, chopped celery, minced onion, organic mayonnaise, and one slice avocado) makes a great lunch.

Dinner options

1. Homemade meatloaf with half a sweet potato and mushroom and green bean salad made a nice filling meal.

2. Try grilled mahi-mahi with steamed broccoli and ½ cup of brown rice.

3. Baked turkey breast with pesto spaghetti squash (you can cook it in microwave for twelve minutes, use fork to thread and then add pesto made with olive oil, parmesan cheese, and pepper) make a flavorful dinner.

4. Try tilapia cooked in vegetable broth with spices, a little white wine, and chopped onions, carrots, and peas with a green salad.

5. Grilled skirt steak with collard greens sautéed in vegetable broth with a little olive oil is easy to make.

6. Try grilled eggplant topped with marinara sauce, baked with once slice of mozzarella cheese. Accompany with yellow and green squash sautéed in broth with garlic and spices.

7. To make quinoa spaghetti primavera, cook pasta as indicated on package; add broccoli, peppers, eggplant, and mushroom sautéed in broth with garlic, seasoned with 1 tablespoon olive oil and parmesan cheese.

8. For lentil stew, cook lentils in marinara sauce with chopped carrots, potatoes, celery, and onions.

9. Try broiled lamb chops marinated in lemon juice, dried mustard, and garlic, with shredded cabbage and carrots dressed in 1 tablespoon olive oil, vinegar, and 1 teaspoon honey.

10. How about seasoned grilled chicken breast with steamed asparagus and broccoli?

11. Try white bean and vegetable soup, a homemade turkey burger, and sautéed collard greens with garlic.

12. For tempeh delight, cut tempeh in cubes and steam-sauté in vegetable broth, garlic, and a little olive oil with mixed vegetables (broccoli, peppers, squash, asparagus, carrots, green beans).

13. Sautéed scallops with roasted vegetables and shredded cabbage salad makes a nice dinner.

14. Roasted chicken with cubed sweet potatoes (dress in olive oil, rosemary, mustard, lemon juice, pepper, oregano and basil before cooking) is nice in the winter.

15. Try broiled salmon dressed with lemon juice, mustard, pepper and a little honey before cooking. Sautéed kale and mushrooms with garlic go with the salmon nicely.

16. You may like grilled lamb chop dressed with cinnamon and dried mustard, accompanied by mashed potatoes with parsley and minced scallions.

17. For a crustless chicken pie, combine 1 cup cooked and chopped chicken mixed with 2 eggs, shredded carrots, peas, minced onions, ½ cup cream, baked on a lightly sprayed oven pan (enough for two), with a mixed salad.

18. Roasted turkey breast with mashed sweet potatoes and green beans are simple and filling.

19. Try brown rice sushi rolls (vegetarian or fish), seaweed salad or green salad with one tablespoon ginger dressing.

20. Try ½ cup brown rice with ½ cup black beans or chickpeas and chopped cooked vegetables in broth and garlic.

Snack options

1. Hummus and celery sticks
2. Turkey and lettuce rolls
3. 1 apple with 1 flat tablespoon organic peanut or almond butter
4. 1 handful raw nuts
5. You can use bars sporadically, but please make sure they only have a few natural ingredients (no more than four or five), like Lara bar or Kind bars.
6. 2 nectarines
7. 1 mandarin orange and 10 raw almonds
8. Half a grapefruit with 1 scoop of cottage cheese seasoned with stevia and cinnamon
9. 1 pear
10. 1 boiled eggs (if you are not eating eggs in your other meals)
11. Half a cup of cherries
12. 1 cup of strawberries with ½ cup plain Kefir, stevia to taste
13. Celery and sticks carrot sticks wrapped in turkey slices
14. large peach
15. 2 kiwis
16. 1 slice Ezekiel bread with a little goat cheese and 1 teaspoon agave
17. Lettuce wrap with hummus
18. ½ cup blueberries with ½ cup plain Kefir
19. 1 tablespoon almond or peanut butter on celery stick
20. Red pepper cut in half topped with hummus
21. ¼ cup raw sunflower or pumpkin seeds

Appendix B: Healthylicious recipes

P art of the process of changing your relationship with food consists of awakening your creative side, relearning to play and have fun, and enjoying all your senses. This is about feeling alive rather than stuffing into numbness. Cooking is a great avenue to change your approach to food. It requires you to slow down and live the process of creation. Food will then acquire a new dimension, it will become your masterpiece, something to enjoy and admire and be proud of as you consciously engage in every bite. After all, you wouldn't gulp down your own Gioconda, would you?

Imagine this scenario: You go shopping and select your food ingredients, picking only the best and only what is in your list. You go home, take off your shoes, put some music (I love Italian music for cooking). You turn into a gourmet food artist, playing and chopping and churning and smelling and dancing, as you cook. Then, while your masterpiece is cooking, you set up a beautiful table. It doesn't matter if you have company or will be eating by yourself, because you are the most important guest. When the time food is ready, you sit down and approach your food creation in awe and respect toward yourself. This whole experience can be a stress reliever, an opportunity to give your mind a break from worries, and fully focus on your playful and creative side. Have a romantic dinner, whether it is with your special other, or by yourself.

On the following pages, you will find some "healthylicious" recipes to spark your imagination and treat yourself to good food. I have collected them over the years. Some of them I learned from family and friends. Some are the product of my playing in the kitchen, and some are contributions from my favorite chefs and restaurants.

For a long time, you have been using food to sooth your emotions. You have tried bingeing on potato chips and already know it doesn't work. So why not try this instead? Channel your energy into preparing and making something healthy and good, and enjoy it, slowly, with intention, with your whole self…loving yourself… Bon Appétit!

Bobe Paulina's Argentinean Chimichurri: Excellent to serve over meat, chicken, or fish

Ingredients:
10 garlic cloves, cut in half lengthwise
1 tablespoon oregano
2 flat teaspoons chili powder
1 tablespoon paprika
8 ounces white vinegar (not apple cider)
24 ounces (3 cups) boiling water

Directions:
Take an empty 1-liter glass bottle and throw inside the garlic, oregano, chili, paprika, and vinegar. Put the handle of a metal teaspoon through bottle opening to avoid glass breaking while you carefully pour in the boiling water. Cover with top or cork and let cool down (can be refrigerated for several weeks). Shake well and pour a little on cooked, grass fed organic steak, chicken, or steamed fish.

My Famous Lentil Stew:

Ingredients:
1 bag lentils
1 chopped onion
1 cup chopped carrots
1 cup diced potato
½ cup chopped celery sticks
½ glass white wine
1 large jar organic tomato sauce
1 small bruschetta spread or tomato pesto paste jar
1 teaspoon raw sugar
sea salt, pepper and Cajun style spices to taste

Directions:
In a large pot, put lentils (previously rinsed) and cover with tomato sauce, bruschetta or pesto spread, and wine. Bring to a boil, add all other ingredients, cover, and reduce heat to low. Cook for one hour or until lentils are tender, adding water as necessary.

Vegetarian Shepherd's Pie

Ingredients:
1 tablespoon olive oil
1 pack firm tofu, drained
1 cup chopped portobello mushrooms
¾ cup medium salsa
½ cup chopped onion
½ teaspoon basil
½ teaspoon oregano
2 cloves garlic, minced
3 cups cooked and mashed sweet potato
salt and pepper
½ tablespoon real butter

Directions:
Heat olive oil in nonstick skillet on medium heat. Add onion and
garlic and stir a few minutes until transparent. Add mashed tofu,
mushrooms, salsa, basil, oregano, salt, and pepper. Stir for several
minutes. Remove from heat.

Spray oven pan and cover bottom with half of the mashed sweet
potato seasoned with salt and pepper and a little bit of butter. Pour
tofu mix over and distribute with fork. Cover with remaining seasoned mashed sweet potato.

Cook in preheated oven at 370 degrees until hot before serving.

Herbed Quinoa:

This is a creation by health food chef Julio Valderrama. He explained, "Quinoa is a superfood because it is nutrient dense. It is a food that I consider a staple in my diet and that I never tire of eating. It's a relatively low calorie food that is wheat, gluten, and cholesterol free, packed with vitamins and minerals. The protein in quinoa is a complete protein since it has the 8 essential amino acids and it is easily digested compared with animal protein. The carbohydrates in quinoa are released slowly, therefore, maintaining the blood sugar level more stable, which in turn keeps you full longer curbing your appetite."

Ingredients:
2 cups Quinoa (dried)
1 bunch finely chopped flat parsley
1 cup finely chopped dill weed
1 cup finely chopped spearmint
1 cup sunflower seeds (toasted)
1 cup chopped scallions
Garlic chopped
1 cube vegetarian bullion,
Olive oil
1/8 cup fresh Lemon juice,
Sea salt to taste
Liquid braggs aminos to taste
A dash of cayenne pepper

Directions:
Soak the quinoa in water for fifteen minutes and then rinse it in a fine colander for a couple of minutes. In a pot big enough for all the ingredients, heat up the olive oil and sauté the garlic and the scallions for a few minutes to release the flavors. Then add 4 cups of filtered water and the rinsed quinoa. Add the bouillon cube and bring to a boil until the water level matches the same level

as the quinoa. Cover and reduce heat to simmer for about ten to fifteen minutes or until fluffy. Remove from heat and let it seat uncovered for five minutes. When it has cooled down a little, add all the chopped herbs and the sunflower seeds. Mix well and season it while mixing with the lemon juice, cayenne pepper, sea salt and liquid brags. Add some olive oil if desired.

Salmon with Spinach & Herb Pesto:

This recipe is a creation by Tania, *chef of her own restaurant, which happens to be one of my favorite places. If you are ever in North Miami Beach and want a gourmet healthy lunch, I highly recommend it.*

2 portions of salmon, 4 to 6 oz. each
Salt & pepper

Place on a sheet and roast in preheated 400 oven for twelve to fifteen minutes.

Meanwhile, in your food processor or blender, mix the following:
1 cup fresh spinach leaves
2 cloves garlic
1 teaspoon dijon mustard
juice of half a lemon
2 tablespoons fresh basil

Slowly add four tbsp extra virgin olive oil and process until smooth. Season to taste and drizzle over salmon.

Marcós Favorite Salad: (Great source of protein and omega-3, courtesy of my friend Adriana)

Ingredients: (Makes four to six servings)
1 can of sardines in fresh water
3 cups of crisp organic lettuce
2 heirloom tomatoes
3 hardboiled eggs cut in quarters
1 small red onion thinly sliced
¼ cup black olives

Vinaigrette:
3 tablespoons of extra-virgin (first cold pressed) olive oil
1 ½ tablespoons of apple cider vinegar
1 tablespoon of freshly squeezed lemon juice
Salt and freshly ground black pepper to taste

To make the vinaigrette, combine the lemon juice and apple cider vinegar in a small bowl. Slowly add the olive oil, whisking constantly until the mixture is smooth. Season with salt and pepper to taste.

To make the salad, combine the lettuce, red onion, and tomatoes in a salad bowl. Pour the dressing over the salad keeping two spoons for later. Garnish with the hardboiled eggs and the sardines. Sprinkle the remaining vinaigrette over the eggs and the sardines, decorate with olives, and serve.

Salmon with a Twist

Ingredients: (Makes four servings)
1 large wild Alaskan salmon fillet
¼ cup agave
juice of 1 fresh lemon
2 tablespoons Dijon mustard
2 minced garlic cloves
Salt and pepper

Directions:
Preheat oven to 375 degrees. Mix agave, mustard, lemon juice, garlic, salt, and pepper. Rub on salmon. Place on oven pan previously sprayed with olive oil and cook until desired consistency, approximately twenty-five to thirty minutes. Serve with steamed vegetables and mixed greens salad.

Almond Butter Soup

Ingredients: (Makes two servings)
1 teaspoon olive oil
½ chopped onion
½ teaspoon curry powder
½ can condensed tomato soup (check ingredients, buy with no added preservatives
 or chemicals)
½ cup vegetable broth, or water
1 tablespoons almond butter
½ tablespoon chopped fresh parsley
Salt and pepper to taste

Directions:
Heat the olive oil in a saucepan and sauté onion until clear and soft, about four minutes. Add curry powder and cook, stirring, for one minute more. Add condensed tomato soup and broth or water. Let simmer. Add almond butter and parsley. Season with salt and pepper. Enjoy hot.

Brown Rice and Lentils with Curry:

Ingredients: (Makes four servings)
1 tablespoon organic butter
1 cup brown rice
4 cups water
1 cup lentils
4 cloves garlic
½ teaspoon cinnamon
A small piece of fresh ginger, peeled and sliced
1 tablespoon curry powder
½ teaspoon unprocessed sea salt
4 scallions

Directions:
Preheat oven to 350 degrees. Melt butter over medium-high heat over stove in a large pot that can then be placed in the oven. Add rice and cook, stirring, until lightly toasted, about 1 ½ minutes. Add curry powder and cook, stirring, about fifteen seconds. Add water. Stir in lentils, chopped garlic cloves, cinnamon stick, ginger, and salt. Bring to a boil. Cover the pot tightly. Put in oven and bake until the rice and lentils are tender and all the water is absorbed, about fifty minutes. Serve garnished with scallions over a bed of spinach.

Rice Pudding: (This is a lactose free dessert.)

Ingredients: (Makes eight servings)
1 cup brown rice
2 cups water
½ teaspoon salt
3 cups rice milk
$1/3$ cup light brown sugar
¼ cup chopped nuts and raisins
½ teaspoon ground cinnamon
1 tablespoon cornstarch
2 ripe bananas, smashed
1 teaspoon vanilla extract

Directions:
Put rice, water, and salt in a saucepan and bring to a boil. Reduce heat to low, cover, and simmer forty-five to fifty minutes, allowing liquid to be absorbed. Add the rice milk, brown sugar, and cinnamon, and allow to simmer. Cook, stirring once in a while, for ten minutes. Mix cornstarch and 1 tablespoon of water in a small bowl until smooth. Add to the pudding. Continue cooking, stirring often, for ten minutes. Remove from heat. Add the mashed bananas and vanilla extract. Cover and refrigerate until very cold. Top with chopped nuts and raisins.

Pie-less Apple Pie:

Ingredients: (Makes one serving)
1 organic apple, peeled and diced
2 tablespoons agave
Cinnamon
juice of ½ fresh lemon
¼ cup raisins

Directions:
Mix all ingredients in a microwave bowl. Microwave on high for one minute. Take a moment to delight in the spirit lifting aroma before eating.

Black Bean Dip:

Ingredients:
1 can black beans, rinsed
½ cup bottled salsa
2 tablespoons fresh lemon juice
1 tablespoon chopped fresh cilantro
1 tablespoon chopped fresh parsley
¼ teaspoon ground cumin
¼ teaspoon oregano
1 bunch of celery sticks, washed and cut in half
Salt and pepper to taste

Directions:
Combine black beans, salsa, lemon juice, parsley, cilantro, salt, pepper and cumin in a blender. Process until smooth. Serve with celery sticks.

Black Bean and Quinoa Delight:

Ingredients: (Makes eight servings)
2 teaspoons extra-virgin olive oil
4 cups cooked quinoa
1 ½ cups chopped onion
2 chopped garlic cloves
1 teaspoon hot Cajun style spice mix
½ teaspoon ground cumin
½ teaspoon dried oregano
2 cans black beans, rinsed
1 cup water
1 tablespoon salsa

Directions:
Heat oil in a saucepan on medium-high heat. Add onion and cook, stirring, four to five minutes. Add garlic and cook, stirring constantly, for thirty seconds. Add spices and cook, stirring, thirty seconds more. Add beans, water, and salsa. Stir until it boils; reduce heat to medium-low and cook, stirring occasionally, for ten minutes. Serve warm over cooked quinoa. You can garnish with steamed vegetables.

Yummy Bok Choy:

Ingredients: (Makes four servings)
3 cups shredded bok choy
1 shredded carrot
$^1/8$ cup rice vinegar
½ tablespoon avocado or olive oil
1 teaspoons raw sugar
1 teaspoons Dijon mustard
Salt to taste
1 chopped scallions

Directions:
Mix vinegar, oil, sugar, mustard, and salt in a bowl until the sugar dissolves. Add bok choy, carrots, and scallions; mix well to coat with the dressing.

Red Cabbage with Mushrooms:

Ingredients: (Makes eight servings)
2 teaspoons olive oil
2 onions, halved lengthwise and thinly sliced
1 head shredded red cabbage
$2/3$ cup vegetable broth
2 teaspoons raw sugar
1 teaspoon caraway seeds
1 can mushrooms
$1/3$ cup apple cider vinegar
Salt and pepper to taste

Directions:
Heat oil in a pot over medium heat. Add onions and cook, stirring often, for five minutes. Add cabbage and cook, stirring occasionally, for five minutes. Add broth, sugar, and caraway seeds; bring to a simmer. Reduce heat to low, cover and cook until the cabbage is very tender, fifteen to twenty minutes. Stir in mushrooms, vinegar, salt, and pepper. Increase heat to medium and cook, uncovered, until most of the liquid has evaporated, five to eight minutes.

Broccoli-Cauliflower Skewers:

Ingredients: (Makes one dozen skewers)
24 broccoli florets
24 cauliflower florets
1 tablespoon reduced-sodium soy sauce
1 tablespoon rice vinegar
1 tablespoon olive oil
1 tablespoon minced fresh ginger
1 tablespoon smooth organic almond butter
1 minced garlic clove garlic
1 teaspoon curry powder
¼ teaspoon salt

Directions:
Boil broccoli and cauliflower for about 3 minutes. Blend soy sauce, vinegar, oil, ginger, almond butter, garlic, curry and salt together. Pour on the florets; gently toss to coat. Let marinate at room temperature for a couple of hours or cover and refrigerate for up to 1 day.
To serve, put 2 broccoli and 2 cauliflower florets onto each skewer. Arrange the skewers on a platter and drizzle with the marinade.

Broccoli Meal in a Soup:

Ingredients: (Makes 6 servings)
1 tablespoon extra-virgin olive oil
1 large chopped onion
1 large sliced carrot
2 stalks chopped celery
1 large potato, peeled and cut in small cubes
2 minced garlic cloves
1 tablespoon whole wheat flour
½ teaspoon dry mustard
1/8 teaspoon cayenne pepper
3 ½ cups vegetable broth
3 cup frozen broccoli florets
1 cup grated cheddar cheese
½ cup plain Kefir
Salt to taste

Directions:
Heat oil in a saucepan over medium-high heat. Cook onion, carrot, and celery, stirring often, five to six minutes. Add potato and garlic; cook, stirring, for two minutes. Add flour, dry mustard, and cayenne; cook, stirring often, for two minutes. Add broth and bring to a boil. Cover and reduce heat to medium. Simmer, stirring occasionally, for ten minutes. Stir in florets; simmer ten more minutes, covered, until the broccoli is tender. Transfer 2 cups of the mix to blender and mash, then return to the pan. Stir in cheddar and kefir; cook over medium heat, stirring, until the cheese is melted and the soup meal is hot. Add salt to taste.

Coconut Coated Tofu with Exotic Salsa:

Ingredients: (Makes four servings)
1 mango, pitted and diced
1-2 jalapenos, preferably red, seeded and minced
1 two-inch piece fresh lemongrass, minced, or 1 teaspoon dried
1 tablespoon chopped fresh basil
1 tablespoon brown sugar
1 tablespoon rice vinegar
¾ teaspoon salt
1/3 cup unsweetened flaked coconut
2 tablespoons flour
2 tablespoons cornstarch
1 package extra-firm water-packed tofu, drained
1 tablespoon olive oil or olive spray

Directions:
Mix mango, jalapenos, lemongrass, basil, brown sugar, vinegar, and
¼ teaspoon salt in a bowl. Mix coconut, flour, and cornstarch in
a dish. Cut the block of tofu lengthwise into 8 thin slices. Pat the
tofu slices dry with a paper towel, sprinkle with the remaining ½
teaspoon salt, and then press both sides of each tofu steak into the
coconut mixture. Heat oil (or spray) in a large nonstick skillet over
medium-high heat. Add tofu steaks and cook until golden brown,
about two minutes per side, lowering heat if necessary to prevent
burning. Serve the tofu with the mango salsa.

Curry Chicken and Quinoa Pasta Salad:

Ingredients: (Makes six servings)

12 ounces quinoa pasta shells

2 tablespoons slivered almonds

1 tablespoon curry powder

½ cup reduced-fat organic mayonnaise

½ cup low-fat plain organic yogurt

1/3 cup mango chutney

1 teaspoon turmeric

¼ teaspoon ground cinnamon

Pinch ground cayenne pepper

2 cups cooked chicken, cut into one-inch pieces

½ cup raisins

½ cup chopped onion

½ cup diced celery

Salt and freshly ground pepper to taste

Directions:

Cook quinoa pasta for ten minutes in a large pot of lightly salted water or until al dente. Drain and rinse. Set aside in large bowl. Toast almonds in a small dry skillet over low heat, stirring constantly, until golden, about two minutes. Transfer to a plate to cool. Return the pan to the stovetop and add curry powder. Toast, stirring constantly, over low heat about thirty seconds. Transfer to a bowl; stir in mayonnaise, yogurt, chutney, turmeric, cinnamon, and ground red pepper. Combine chicken, raisins, onion, celery, and the reserved pasta in a large bowl. Add the dressing and mix well. Garnish with the toasted almonds.

Edamame Stew:

Ingredients: (Makes four servings)
3 cups frozen shelled edamame, thawed
1 tablespoon extra-virgin olive oil
1 large chopped onion
1 large zucchini, diced
2 tablespoons minced garlic
2 teaspoons ground cumin
1 teaspoon ground coriander
1/8 teaspoon cayenne pepper, or to taste
1 can Italian diced tomatoes
¼ cup chopped fresh mint
3 tablespoons lemon juice

Directions:
Boil edamame and until tender, four to five minutes or according to package directions. Drain. Heat oil in a large saucepan over medium heat. Add onion and cook, covered, stirring occasionally, until starting to soften, about three minutes. Add zucchini and cook, covered, until the onions are starting to brown, about three minutes more. Add garlic, cumin, coriander, and cayenne, and cook, stirring, about thirty seconds. Stir in tomatoes and bring to a boil; reduce heat to a simmer and cook until slightly reduced, about five minutes. Stir in the edamame and cook until heated through, about two minutes more. Remove from the heat and stir in mint and lemon juice.

Fennel, Cabbage and Sweet Potato Stew:

Ingredients:
1 tablespoon extra-virgin olive oil, divided
1 bag shredded cabbage
1 large bulb fennel, thinly sliced
1 small onion, sliced
1 teaspoon garlic powder
½ teaspoon fennel seed
½ teaspoon ground pepper
2 cups cooked cubed sweet potato (you can use canned or frozen)
1 cup vegetable broth
¼ cup rice vinegar
1 tablespoon brown mustard

Directions:
Add oil to the pan and heat over medium heat. Add cabbage, sliced fennel, onion, garlic powder, fennel seed, and pepper, and cook, stirring often, for three minutes. Add sweet potatoes and cook, stirring occasionally, until the potatoes are heated through, two to four minutes. Add broth, vinegar and mustard and stir until the mustard is incorporated; bring to a simmer, cover, reduce heat to medium-low and cook until the vegetables are tender, seven to ten minutes, adding more broth if necessary.

Skillet Quinoa shells with Chard & White Beans:

Ingredients: (Makes six servings)
½ tablespoon extra-virgin olive oil
½ package of quinoa shells, cooked al dente and drained
1 onion, thinly sliced
4 cloves garlic, minced
½ cup water
6 cups chopped chard leaves (about 1 small bunch) or spinach
1 can diced tomatoes with Italian seasonings
1 can white beans, rinsed
¼ teaspoon ground pepper
½ cup shredded part-skim organic mozzarella cheese
¼ cup finely shredded Parmesan cheese

Directions:
Heat oil in nonstick skillet over medium heat. Add onion and cook, stirring, over medium heat, for two minutes. Stir in garlic and water. Cover and cook until the onion is soft, four to six minutes. Add chard (or spinach) and cook, stirring, one to two minutes. Stir in tomatoes, beans, and pepper, and bring to a simmer. Stir in the pasta and sprinkle with mozzarella and Parmesan. Cover and cook until the cheese is melted and the sauce is hot, about three minutes.

Mushroom Pasta:

Ingredients: (Serves four)
8 ounces portobello mushrooms, sliced
8 ounces quinoa noodles, cooked
1 ½ cups vegetable broth
1 medium onion, finely chopped
3 tablespoons flour
3 tablespoons olive oil
1 ½ cups fat-free organic sour cream
¼ cup parsley, chopped
Salt and pepper

Directions:
Mix the sour cream and flour together in a small bowl until smooth.
Set aside. In a large skillet, sauté the onion in the olive oil over low
heat until soft. Turn the heat up to medium-high and add the mushrooms. Sauté until the mushrooms brown. Transfer the mushroom
mixture to a bowl. Turn the heat up to high and add the broth to
the skillet. Bring to a boil and reduce the liquid by 30 percent. Set
the heat to low and add the mushrooms and onions. Add sour cream
and flour mixture to skillet, stirring well. Add parsley. Season with
salt and pepper to taste. Serve over quinoa noodles.

Tofuloaf

Ingredients: (Serves twelve)
1 package firm tofu
1 cup brown rice, cooked
2 cups Italian bread crumbs
1 medium carrot, finely chopped
2 medium celery stalks, finely chopped
1 small onion, finely chopped
1 cup walnuts, finely chopped
2 teaspoons Dijon mustard
3 tablespoons liquid amino acids (or soy sauce)
¼ cup barbecue sauce plus a little more
¼ teaspoon black pepper

Directions:
Preheat oven to 350 degrees. Blend the tofu in a food processor until smooth. Set aside. Mix the brown rice, carrot, celery, onion, walnuts, and bread crumbs together in a large bowl. Add the tofu purée, liquid amino acids, mustard, ¼ cup barbecue sauce, and black pepper to the rice mixture and combine well. Spray a 5x9-inch baking pan with nonstick cooking spray. Transfer the mixture to the baking pan and top with the extra barbecue sauce. Place the dish in the preheated oven and bake for one hour. Let stand for ten to fifteen minutes after baking. Slice and serve with additional barbecue sauce if desired.

Cranberry Turkey:

Ingredients: (Makes four servings)
4 medium fennel bulbs, thickly sliced
2 tablespoons olive oil
½ teaspoon chopped fresh thyme
1 teaspoon sea salt
¾ teaspoon ground pepper
4 turkey cutlets
1 cup cranberry juice
¼ cup vegetable broth or water
1 teaspoon cornstarch

Directions:
Preheat oven to 450°F. Toss fennel, 1 tablespoon oil, chopped thyme and ¼ teaspoon each salt and pepper in a bowl. Spread on a baking sheet. Roast, stirring a few times, until tender and golden, about a half hour. Meanwhile, sprinkle both sides of turkey with the remaining salt and pepper. Heat the remaining oil in a large skillet over medium-high heat. Add the turkey and cook until browned, one to three minutes per side. Transfer to a plate. Add cranberry juice to the pan; bring to a boil. Boil, stirring often, until reduced to ¼ cup, six to ten minutes. Mix together broth (or water) and cornstarch; add to the pan and cook, stirring constantly, until thickened, about fifteen seconds. Reduce heat to medium, return the turkey and any accumulated juices to the pan, turning to coat with sauce, and cook for one minute. To serve, top roasted fennel with turkey and sauce.

Brussels Sprouts with Shallots:

Ingredients: (Makes six half-cup servings)
12 small shallots
1 tablespoons extra-virgin olive oil
1 pounds Brussels sprouts
1 teaspoon sea salt

Directions:
Preheat oven to 375° F. Place peeled shallots on a large sheet of parchment paper; sprinkle ½ tablespoon oil over the top. Seal the packet and bake until the shallots are tender, about forty-five minutes. Remove from packet and set aside to cool. Meanwhile, remove the outer leaves from Brussels sprouts and trim the stems. Cut the sprouts in half. Place the shallots and Brussels sprouts in a roasting pan. Toss with the remaining oil and salt. Roast, tossing a few times during cooking, until the Brussels sprouts are tender and lightly browned, about forty minutes.

Sautéed Kale:

Ingredients:
1 tablespoon extra-virgin olive oil
1 pound kale, ribs removed, coarsely chopped
½ cup water
2 cloves minced garlic
¼ teaspoon cayenne pepper
2-3 teaspoons red-wine vinegar
¼ teaspoon unprocessed sea salt

Directions:
Heat oil in a pot over medium heat. Add kale and cook, tossing, until bright green, about one minute. Add water, reduce heat to medium-low, cover and cook, stirring occasionally, until the kale is tender, about fifteen minutes. Push kale to one side, and cook garlic for thirty seconds. Remove from heat. Stir in vinegar, cayenne, and salt.

French Riviera Tofu:

Ingredients: (Makes two servings)
1 pack extra-firm, water-packed tofu, drained
1 tablespoon cornstarch
1 tablespoon whole wheat flour
Salt and pepper to taste
1 tablespoon extra-virgin olive oil
¾ cup vegetable broth
2-3 tablespoons red-wine vinegar
2 tablespoons chopped olives
2 tablespoons chopped pitted dates

Directions:
Cut tofu crosswise into four ½-inch-thick slices. Pat with paper towels to remove excess moisture. Whisk cornstarch, flour, salt, and pepper in a dish. Heat oil in a nonstick skillet over medium-high heat. Dredge the tofu in the cornstarch mixture. Add the tofu to the pan and cook, turning once, until crispy and golden, two to four minutes per side. Transfer to a plate and cover to keep warm. Add broth and vinegar to the pan; bring to a simmer, stirring often. Add olives, dates, and pepper, and simmer until heated through, one to two minutes. To serve, spoon the sauce over the tofu.

Warm Beet Salad:

Ingredients: (Makes four servings)
8 cups baby spinach
1 tablespoon extra-virgin olive oil
1 cup thinly sliced red onion
2 plum tomatoes, chopped
2 tablespoons sliced olives
2 tablespoons chopped fresh parsley
1 clove minced garlic
2 cups cooked beet slices
2 tablespoons balsamic vinegar
¼ teaspoon salt
¼ teaspoon freshly ground pepper

Directions:
Heat oil in a nonstick skillet over medium heat. Add onion and cook, stirring, until starting to soften, about two minutes. Add tomatoes, olives, parsley, and garlic, and cook, stirring, until the tomatoes begin to break down, about three minutes. Add beets, vinegar, salt, and pepper, and cook, stirring, until the beets are heated through, about one minute more. Place the beet mixture over spinach on a plate and mix to combine. Serve warm.

Appendix C: Supplements

There is much controversy around the need or even useful-ness of taking supplements and vitamins. My suggestion is to get information from trusted sources, check with your health care provider, and then make an educated decision.

Some professionals say it is a waste of time and money, and others say they are indispensable. Probably the truth is somewhere in between.

Most fruit and vegetables we eat nowadays come from faraway lands, and have been sitting in warehouses, trucks, planes, and ultimately food stores for many days, usually a few weeks. This is so, even when we buy at some health food stores. By the time we buy our food, it has probably lost a great deal of its enzymes and properties.

I personally chose to take some supplements on which I have found plentiful serious research evidencing results and safety. Here is the list of what I personally take, in case it helps you do your own research and make a decision:

1. A good multi-vitamin and anti-oxidant formula made from whole foods (not synthetic, free of chemicals)
2. Extra vitamin C (How come we forget a Nobel Prize was awarded for discovering its effects on the immune system?)
3. A sub-lingual liquid B vitamin complex (A lot of good stud-ies showing mood balancing properties, plus, it is very im-portant for vegetarians, who are often deficient in B-12.); I take it in the morning because it gives me an energy boost.
4. Chia seed: it has amazing quantities of Omega 3s from veg-etable source (One tablespoon contains almost 3000 mg

and it also provides fiber.); many experts recommend it to prevent inflammation, boost memory and focus, manage weight, and balance mood. Fish oil is also a great source of Omega 3s. I *don't* take it because I often eat sardines, salmon, and other fish rich in this essential fatty acids. If you don't eat enough of these fish and decide to take it as a supplement, chose a brand that has been purified from PCVs, mercury, and other heavy *metals*, and where the major components are EPA and DHA (real Omega 3s), instead of filler oils like soybean oil.

4. Vitamin D; most health practitioners now recommend it and there is much research pointing to its strengthening effect on the immune system, preventing cancer and much more.

5. A good plant based digestive enzyme, to compensate for the loss of living enzymes in food nowadays

6. Alpha Lipoic Acid: a great anti-oxidant and liver protector

Q&A with Expert Contributions

I n this section, you will find helpful answers generously provided
by talented and respected experts in different fields related to
women's health and weight management.

Janet Konefal, PhD., M.P.H., is the assistant dean of the
University of Miami, Miller School of Medicine. She is in charge
of the Integrative Medicine Department, and a pioneer in the field.
This is what she had to say in reference to weight management:

What is the role of integrative medicine?

Integrative medicine is a combination of conventional and comple-
mentary medicine that focuses on partnership among the health
care providers and the individual patient. A major focus of comple-
mentary medicine is now clinical nutrition. As research continues
to explore how nutrition plays a role in our physical, mental,
emotional, and spiritual well-being, it will continue to move into
mainstream medicine and become the first line of medicine.

How can integrative medicine help women deal with weight management?

Focusing only on weight management without considering how this affects the health of the person can be irresponsible and lead to unwanted
results. Being healthy includes weight management. Unless you are one
of the those lucky individuals with a set of genes that allows you to be
careless about your life style and still maintain your health, you, like
most of us, require due diligence to maintain your health and, therefore, weigh in within a healthy range. An integrative medicine approach
allows you to find and apply what works for you.

What is in your opinion the biggest challenge nowadays for women when it comes to maintaining a healthy weight?

Our food supply is so full of processed foods that unhealthy eating is partly a social disease and sometimes we actually make fun of people who go out of their way to eat healthy. The National Cancer Institute recommends eating four to nine servings of fruits and vegetables a day. This is very difficult to do in many work places. Then we tend to oversize our portions. The average refined sugar intake in America is over 180 pounds per person per year and most of it is already in the prepared foods. There are so many additives in our food that have not been tested for any long-term effects that the National Medical Advisory Council has suggested an association between these toxins and our ever increasing plague of chronic diseases. We serve some of the unhealthiest food selections to our children and to our sick via our schools and hospitals. The biggest challenge is awareness and then applying the awareness to the choices made. Women cannot only help themselves, but can take the lead in helping our communities become healthy.

If you could give one piece of advice for Princess Sandra, what would that be?

Two suggestions: One, eat mindfully, eat with your future in mind. Two, ask for specific support from friends and family. Think about what each person around you could do to support you and then ask for this support. For example, if someone at work is always offering you sugary eats, ask them not to do this anymore. Here's a little exercise you may find helpful. Create an image of a healthy you in your future. Make this image of yourself as you want to be. Not just at the weight you want to achieve, but including all the behaviors that support you being healthy at the desired weight. Create lots of detail about this future you. Make the image real for yourself.

Include the emotional resources and see yourself surrounded by the support you need.

'ᵀᴴᏬ 'ᵀᴴᏬ 'ᵀᴴᏬ

Etti Ben-Zion is a doctor in Holistic Nutrition, specializing in juice fasting and detox. This is what she had to say regarding the use of juice fasting and weight management:

What is the correlation between toxins and excess weight? Why is detoxing so important? What is the best way for detoxing in your opinion?

A juice fast is a great way to promote health issues, detoxify your body, and deal with disease symptoms. Fortunately, this healthful practice also causes a very noticeable loss of fat as well. Juice fasting for weight loss is a great way to keep your body at a healthy weight.

It makes sense that this detoxification diet will also relieve you of unwanted body fat because many toxins are found in the fat cells. By eliminating the fat, the toxins are released into the body so that they can be eliminated through the typical procedures, such as urination or through the lungs. This is why juice fasting gives you energy and provides better overall health.

By unlocking the pure nutrients from fruits and vegetables, a juice extractor gives you the opportunity to obtain pure energy from the juice, leaving your body to release toxins from various sources. Depending on the amount of weight to be lost, the person's level of activity, and their overall metabolism, a person can lose over one pound a day on this fasting regime.

Juice fasting is one of the most healthy ways to shed unwanted pounds that encumber you and harbor toxic substances. However,

<u>there are people who should not try this form of dieting. Pregnant and nursing mothers, people with diabetes or other blood sugar issues, people with liver or kidney disease, or other chronic conditions should discuss any dietary changes with their doctor before starting.</u>

Side effects from juice fasting can include headaches, fatigue, hypoglycemia, constipation, acne, body odor, and bad breath. If you have dizziness, blood pressure problems, unexpected weight loss, vomiting, diarrhea, or worsening symptoms for long-term issues, stop juice fasting and get checked out by a medical professional. Most people do well with the fast, but some conditions may be aggravated by it.

Juice fasting for weight loss is a great way for a healthy person to eliminate unhealthy and unwanted pounds. By following common sense rules and easing your body in and out of the fast, you can lose weight while eliminating toxins from your system. (Author's note: Please do not attempt any form of fasting, including juice fasting without supervision by a competent health practitioner)

If you had one piece of advice for Princess Sandra, what would that be?

My advice for Princess Sandra would be ultimately you can eat and drink and be gorgeous if you have sound loving relationship with yourself. Give yourself mega doses of Vitamin L—love—every day!! Fill your LOVE-BUCKET with simple gestures that will fulfill you, like taking a walk on the beach, taking a yoga class, reading a book, soaking in a bubble bath. Take time-out to go within and LOVE the most important person in your life, which is YOU!!!

TH TH TH

Mano (Mariano) Ardissone, E.R.Y.T., M.M.Q., is founder and director of Ayama Yoga Center, Aventura, FL, where he teaches yoga and practices Chinese Medical Qigong. He is also a traditional Reiki Master and a Transformational Breath Work facilitator. These are his answers regarding weight management and yoga:

Why is it so unusual to find an overweight person in a yoga class?

It is usually hard to find an overweight person in a yoga class because most overweight people try to avoid exposing themselves to others who they think may be fitter or in better shape than they are. There is the general misconception that to attend a yoga class someone needs to be already flexible and/or fit. Overweight people usually have to deal with both of these obstacles, in addition to the psycho-emotional related issues that limit how they see themselves, how they feel others see them, and how they choose to relate to other people in public settings. Yoga classes are for all and more so for those who feel either not fit or not flexible enough; however the ultimate goal of yoga is not to look good, but rather to feel go, so that then we can focus on a truly spiritual pursuit.

How can Eastern practices help to manage weight?

Eastern practices, such as yoga and Qigong, are very powerful and transformative tools that overweight people can utilize to help re-vert the process that led them to their condition. As we know, the human being is made of different layers. In a simplified format, we can speak of the physical, the energetic, the mental-emotional, and the spiritual layers. Each of them are as real as the air we breathe and for a person to be in overall health there needs to be balance within each layer, between each layer, and between the self as a whole and it surroundings. From an eastern perspective, the root cause for being overweight may be located in any of these layers. Thus, it is most effective when dealing with a case of obesity to find that layer where the imbalance originated. Only in this way true healing can take place, otherwise we would be treating the symptoms but not the "disease." Nonetheless, the human being is so intelligent in its makeup, that although it may take longer, there are certain practices such as yoga and Qigong that will slowly help rebalance ALL layers of the self, bringing back harmony to the individual. General group practices will surely help with this, but it would be more effective if it were possible to work individually with the person to create a customized program.

If you had one piece of advice for Princess Sandra, what would that be?

If I had one moment to share with Princess Sandra, I would tell her that accepting herself and loving herself as she is should be her utmost concern. I would advise her to write on her bathroom mirror the affirmation "I love myself" and read it three times every time she sees it. Finally, I would advise her to seek professional help to correct her diet, to include yoga as a daily practice, and to understand the ultimate reason why she may be overweight

ᏨᎾ ᏨᎾ ᏨᎾ

Emmanuela Wolloch, MD, fellow, American College of OB/GYN, is a French gynecologist specializing in hormones. This is her point of view:

How can hormonal imbalances be detected and how do they relate to weight management?

In my gynecological practice, weight management is one of the manifestations of hormonal imbalance. A woman's ovaries produce estrogen every day until menopause. They also produce progesterone in the second part of their menstrual cycle right after ovulation. Less than optimal progesterone levels such as those observed in PMS or peri-menopause will create hormonal imbalance and weight management issues. The solution is to test progesterone levels through a blood test or a saliva test and supplement with natural progesterone, orally or transdermally.

A woman's thyroid can also be a source of weight gain if the production of thyroid hormones decreases to a very low level as detected through a blood test. Prescribing thyroid supplements will reestablish normal blood level of thyroid hormones, enabling optimum metabolism and proper weight management. Some patients may be concerned that taking hormones will make them gain weight. This might be based on the experience many women have with birth-control pills. But taking low doses of natural and balanced hormones will not be a source of extra weight.

᛭ᛏᚻ ᛏᚻ ᛏᚻ᛭

Julio Valderrama is a health food expert and restaurant owner in Miami. His involvement with natural foods started twenty years ago. This is his opinion on food and weight management:

How did you develop a habit of choosing healthy foods?

I had a desire to optimize my physical existence on this planet. Eating healthy does not require a big effort, but rather a gradual obvious understanding that we are not meant to eat for pleasure but for nutritional purposes. This is not to say that we cannot enjoy what we eat. It has become clear to me over the years that we have learned to chose what we put into our bodies with our thoughts and emotions instead of letting our bodies speak to us about the right choices. This process of deciding what to eat should be the same regardless of how slim or overweight one might be.

If you had one piece of advice to Princess Sandra, what would that be?

If you decide to choose a diet of natural and wholesome foods that are not processed, full of fresh fruits and raw vegetables that are packed with nutrients, and if you make those choices a lifestyle, then you don't need to worry about counting calories, fat grams, fiber content, or how many carbohydrates you take each day because the math has already been figured out by the Creator who has created all the wonderful foods that nature provides.

Useful Resources

Here is a list of websites and organizations you may find useful:

My website: you will find plenty of articles and useful information on weight management, diet and nutrition, psychology and hypnosis.
www.cre8yourhealth.com

Crohn's and Colitis Foundation of America
www.ccfa.org

Hippocrates Institute—offers great raw food based programs:
www.hippocratesinst.org

Local Harvest (Community Supported Agriculture)
Find fresh local produce in your area
www.localharvest.org/csa/

Mayo Clinic (Health and Drug Information)
www.mayoclinic.com/health/drug-information/DrugHerbIndex

National Center for Complimentary and Alternative Medicine
List of herbs, research, known side effects, and important information
www.nccam.nih.gov/health/herbsataglance.htmNational Organic Program
www.ams.usda.gov/nop

Slow Food Movement
www.slowfoodusa.org

Support groups for eating disorders
www.eatingdisordersanonymous.org
www.oa.org

The Celiac Disease Foundation
www.celiac.org

About the Author

Patricia Rotsztain Frost was born in Argentina in 1964. She has a Master's Degree in Science from the School of Psychological Studies of Nova Southeastern University, Fl., and is a Licensed Mental Health Counselor, Certified Hypnotherapist (National Guild of Hypnotists), and PhDabd in Natural Health.

She has a private practice where she helps clients individually and in groups, in person and online. Patricia is the director of the Integrative Wellness Forum and creator of the HEAL Program for a Healthy Empowered Assertive Life. She lectures and presents workshops and seminars for public and private organizations, and presented at the International Integrative Medicine Symposium of the University of Miami in 2010.

"I hope you have enjoyed this book and will find it useful in your road towards a new healthy, fit and empowered You.
If you have questions, please email me at patri.frost@gmail.com, and remember to visit my website at www.cre8yourhealth.com for useful information on weight management, psychology and hypnosis.
Your well-being is your birthright and my mission"

Patricia Rotsztain Frost, LMHC, PhDabd

Secret #1:

The scale is not your enemy; it's your copilot.
Pg. 1

Secret #2:

Exercise...your right to be fit
Pg. 11

Secret #3:

Keep your cortisol in check.
Manage stress and sleep well.
Pg. 21

Secret #4:

Hormones rule
Pg. 33

Secret #5:

Natural vs. processed
Pg. 43

Secret #6:

Be like the ameba,
stay away from what's bad
Pg. 61

Appendix B:
Healthylicious recipes
Pg. 129

🍓 **Bobe Paulina's Argentinean Chimichurri**
Pg. 131

🍓 **My Famous Lentil Stew**
Pg. 132

🍓 **Vegetarian Shepherd's Pie**
Pg. 133

🍓 **Herbed Quinoa**
Pg. 135

🍓 **Salmon with Spinach & Herb Pesto**
Pg. 136

🍓 **Marco's Favorite Salad**
Pg. 137

🍓 **Salmon with a Twist**
Pg. 138

🍓 **Almond Butter Soup**
Pg. 139

🍓 **Brown Rice and Lentils with Curry**
Pg. 140

Appendix C:
Supplements

Q&A with Expert Contributions

Useful Resources

About the Author